Visit this book on the World-Wide Web

http://lifeforce.iinet.net.au

All profits from the sale of this book will go to cancer support, to enable their wonderful teams' to continue with the work of helping people from all walks of life - their families and friends - in dealing with cancer.

As the Cancer Support Association motto so aptly states:
CANCER IS A WORD ..... NOT A SENTENCE!

Cover: Cascade Falls, near Pemberton, Western Australia

What people are saying about 'Living Simply with Cancer'...

'Thank you for sharing your beautiful book... simple in its message... so powerful in its meaning and a contribution for so many...'

Julie Stafford, Ballarat, Victoria
Best Selling author; 'Stepping Out', 'Taste of Life' Cookbooks & 'Juicing for Health'

'We... found it (the book) informative, sensible and reassuring. It is the sort of book that should be read by everyone - not just cancer patients.'

I&J Garthwaite, Duncraig, Western Australia

'I am now on a vegetarian and fruit juice diet, and have replaced margarine and butter with avocado!... Thanks for your talk (to the Singapore Cancer Society) and beautiful book...'

Katherine Teng, Singapore

'It is a fantastic book, easy to read and understand...I thoroughly enjoyed it...'

Rosalind Petersen, Booragoon, Western Australia
WA Sports Model of the Year '97

'The shocking realisation that after two major operations, my melanoma had once again developed, I did not know where to turn. I was only 32 and my wife was three months pregnant with our first child. Devastated, I realised I needed help. I read a book by Ross Taylor called 'Living Simply with Cancer'. It was from this point that my life changed. Now officially in remission, I firmly believe that 'Living Simply with Cancer' assisted me not only with my healing process, it has provided me with the tools I need to enjoy what is a very wonderful world.'

Darren Cooper, Joondalup, Western Australia

'Tender, graceful and an easy-to-read approach. Many thanks for sharing yourself and your journey.'

Lucille Hanley
Perth, Western Australia

LIVING simply
 WITH **CANCER**

..... *a guide to dealing with cancer.*

by

ROSS TAYLOR

~ CONTENTS ~

	Foreword	2
	Acknowledgment	4
Chapter 1	Introduction	6
Chapter 2	A Personal Experience	9
Chapter 3	What can I do to help myself?	12
	- Getting started	13
	- Your relationship with the oncologist	14
	- Someone to talk with	18
	- Cancer, stress and the immune system	18
	- The Carer, a spouse's perspective	20
	- A mothers experience	22
	- Feeling for the Family	24
	- Men are not Mountains	25
Chapter 4	Conventional Treatments	26
	- Chemotherapy	26
	- Radiotherapy	29
	- The Decision to Undertake Chemo & Radiotherapy	30
Chapter 5	Creating the 'healing' environment	32
	- Four key areas	33
Chapter 6	Diet (Inner Body Functions)	35
	- What Foods Are Best	36
	- Potassium & Sodium	38
	- What Foods To Consume	39
	- A Choice To Make	41
	- A Special Look At Juicing	44

	- What Juices Are Best	47
	- How To Make Fresh Juices	49
	- Body Cleansing Programme	50
	- Juices – Other Combinations	51
	- Juices – For Specific Disorders	52
	- Fruits	53
	- A Typical Daily Diet	56
Chapter 7	Meditation (The power of a peaceful mind)	60
	- The 'Monkey Mind'	62
	- Just How Powerful Is Our Mind?	63
	- Creative Visualisation	64
	- The Greatest Test	65
	- Getting Started	66
	- Guided Meditation	69
	- 'Mis'-Guided Meditation	69
	- Transcendental Meditation (T.M.)	70
Chapter 8	Physical Fitness (The Outer Body)	73
Chapter 9	Spiritual (A Higher Power)	76
	- The emotional connection	77
Chapter 10	Reiki - Ancient art of energy transfer	78
	- A Brief History	79
	- Our first 'Reiki' experience	80
Chapter 11	Vitamins	82
	- A note about Selenium	83
Chapter 12	Looking ahead	85
Chapter 13	Sources and References	88

Credits

Publishers	Wesprint Holdings Pty Ltd 356a Rokeby Road Subiaco, Western Australia 6008
Type preparation	Kathy Kelly Yong Mee Yuen Diana Cameron
Illustrations	Tony Hardy Individual Images, Greenwood, Western Australia
Proof Readings	Dr Van Ikin, University of Western Australia Marjory Ikin Jennie Parnell
Support Assistance	Andre Malan Fran Spencer Bill Baker, Cancer Support International, Canada
Advertising	Marketforce Advertising, Hay Street, West Perth.
Transport	Courier Australia, Walters Drive, Herdsman, WA.

National Library of Australia Reference:
ISBN 0 646 30875 0
First edition published November 1996
Second edition published June 1998

Front cover photograph with the generous permission of Norm Kelly Photography, and author's photograph with the courtesy of Greg Burke, Duncraig, Western Australia.

© Copyright Ross Taylor 1996, 1998

No part of this book may be reproduced without the consent of the copyright holder.

In memory of Betty

*Who passed over in 1991
following her long journey
with cancer*

– FOREWORD –

by Olivia Newton-John

In 1992 I had just released my 18th album called 'Back to Basics' and I was very honoured to have been named Goodwill Ambassador for the United Nations Environment Programme and spokesperson for the Colette Chuda Environment Fund, named in honour of my best friend's daughter, who had died from cancer the previous year. Then I was diagnosed with cancer!

For the next two years I would suffer the nightmare of facing cancer, including eight months of chemotherapy, plus reconstructive surgery.

Like most people when first diagnosed with cancer, my whole world was effectively turned upside down. My daughter Chloe, was only six years of age, and the thought of possibly not seeing her grow up was terrifying.

Until this time I had little understanding of the drugs used in chemotherapy and what effect they would have on me during treatment. This was to be a time of not only getting to understand the new world of a cancer patient, but also a time to reassess my own life and values.

It was in Australia while visiting the ladies wash-room, that an unknown woman came up to me and explained that she had suffered from breast cancer... 18 years previously. I can remember thinking, 'wow, you can survive that long!' That experience was really important to me and highlighted the importance of seeking support and counselling.

Foreword

On reflection, my experience of surviving breast cancer was in some ways a gift. One of the gifts was the ability to focus less on 'Oh my God, what if...?' and learning to live simply for today, being happy that I'm here right now and being in the moment. I also learned the power of positive thinking.

If you have just been diagnosed don't 'freak out' at the word cancer. Remember my friend 18 years on? The Cancer Support Association in Perth, Australia has a beautiful and powerful saying, 'Cancer is a word, not a (death) sentence'.

There are many things you can do to help in your recovery from cancer. Find a specialist with whom you can feel comfortable, and seek out a support group where you can meet people who have travelled the cancer path.

By simply changing your diet to a high intake of fruit, vegetables and grains, by reducing stress through the gentle art of meditation or prayer, or practicing your own faith (I use 'TM' or Transcendental Meditation and it's wonderful) and seeking out support, you can have a major effect on your general wellbeing, and often your prognosis.

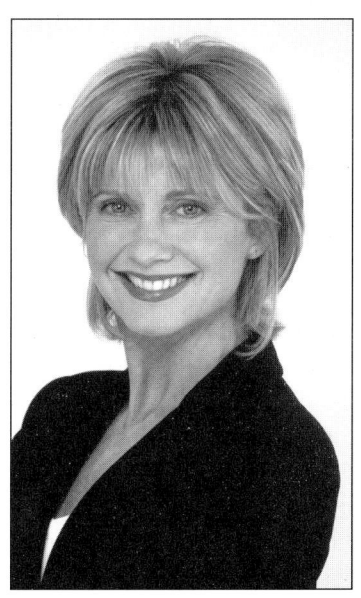

When I first read Ross Taylor's 'Living Simply with Cancer' I was so very pleasantly surprised, for here was a book full of positive, straight-forward information on the practical and the spiritual solutions for people living with cancer.

This book is Ross' second edition of 'Living Simply with Cancer' and so much of what he writes about I have experienced, and I think that anyone dealing with the early stages of discovery of cancer, or going through the process, will find this book very helpful.

It is a quick and easy read, with healing methods for the inner and outer body, both dietary and spiritual. I highly recommend 'Living Simply with Cancer' to you!

– ACKNOWLEDGMENT –

It is with great humility that I acknowledge the wonderful contribution many people continue to make to not only my ongoing good health and personal growth, but also to the continuing success of this book.

Many people from around the world have contacted me and our friends seeking support and guidance, plus commenting on the assistance they have been given from reading 'Living simply with Cancer.' For this I say thank you, for there can be no greater reward than to know that in some small way we have contributed to improving someone's prognosis and/or quality of life, and at the same time raising funds for cancer support.

In the first edition of this book I acknowledged a number of people and they continue to provide me with enormous strength and encouragement. In particular, my friends at the weekly support meetings at the Cancer Support Association are often inspirational, usually humorous, and always open and honest about themselves and the group.

To Cathy, Gerri, Angela, Pam, Denis and Margaret who together edited this edition, my thanks. And of course Doreen, whose wonderful idea it was to include the illustrations 'to make people laugh' my sincere gratitude.

My wife Katherine and I continue to grow together, and her ongoing support and incredible intuition constantly amazes me! I also reflect on the support given to me by some of our

Acknowledgment

long standing friends, their names too many to list here in detail. But I do acknowledge Marie Rome and Margaret Roeterdink who during those first few terrible months quietly went about seeking out information and suitable reading material which would inevitably guide me along this new and exciting path.

Since 1997 I have been working closely with our friends at Lapis Lazuli Light Total Health Library in Singapore and Kuala Lumpur, Malaysia and have been privileged to speak to a number of groups in South East Asia on a regular basis during my visits to the region.

It was during a recent talk in Penang, Malaysia that I was to meet Professor Chris Teo who has undertaken wonderful work through the use of Chinese herbs and the use of 'living' foods. During our discussions it emerged that we shared a common vision, that being to one day create a world-wide support group, called Cancer Care International, which would provide a level of quality support equal to that which we are so fortunate to enjoy here in Perth, Western Australia.

Above the door of every cancer centre will be these words which have been adapted from Professor Teo's vision:

> 'May a thousand flowers bloom,
> and let them shower love and care to all those in need'.

It would be remiss of me not to mention the contribution from Olivia Newton-John. Olivia and her asssistant Dana Sharpe have been so understanding and supportive in completing the Foreword to this book despite a very busy schedule. You are very special people!

And here in Australia, the assistance and support from Channel Nine's Tina Altieri was typical of a person that gives so much to the community. Thanks Tina!

What also remains for us to do is to encourage the medical profession to embrace a holistic approach to healing. This will be an enormous task, but it can be achieved as many enlightened doctors are seeing the immense benefit for their patients in combining the best of medical knowledge with sensible and proven complementary treatments.

Ross Taylor
June 1998

CHAPTER 1

– INTRODUCTION –

The purpose of this book is, hopefully to help people and their families overcome the initial trauma of being diagnosed with cancer, and to take control of their lives by simple yet effective actions.

It would be quite wrong to say that there is some magical cure for cancer - the whole subject is very complex indeed. There is, however, much one can do to significantly improve their quality of life and in many instances enjoy a full and long life filled with a new awareness and enjoyment.

Today, the range of treatments and the arguments for and against them is wide and varied. Some 'experts' will tell you that conventional treatment is harmful, while others will argue that 'alternative' methods such as meditation, diet and energy healing just give false hope.

A 'partnership' approach to healing and treatment would not only improve the health of millions of people, but would also save our Western medical care systems from breaking down due to the massive costs of treating people for the symptoms rather than the cause of their particular illness.

Surely something is wrong with a system that provides, for example, a middle-aged executive with endless supplies of drugs to lower blood pressure without considering why

Chapter 1

it occurred in the first place. To 'bombard' a patient suffering from stress and headaches with 'Valium' and other relaxants, rather than to teach them relaxation techniques and meditation to reduce the stress in the first place, simply leads to higher medical costs and often poorer health.

The situation with cancer is no different. I am often shocked to hear cancer specialists refer to 'complementary' therapies as 'quackery' and 'witchcraft', citing that there is no firm evidence to suggest that diet, meditation and physical activities, for example, will help fight cancer.

Even if we assumed for a moment that the doctors, and the 'medical model' were correct, I am sure most doctors would agree that - putting cancer aside - these activities would provide their patients with significantly improved GENERAL health... so why don't they discuss and recommend these to their patients?

My belief is that both 'conventional' and 'alternative' treatments have a role to play. I can always recall listening to one of the C.S.A.'s facilitators, Cathy Brown, as she once outlined her vision for the future...

'One can only dream and hope that one day all groups will work together, in harmony to complement each other for the benefit of those with cancer.'

Fortunately, the work of people such as Dr. Ian Gawler (the Gawler Foundation) is slowly being acknowledged by the medical establishment.

We believe that 'alternative' therapies will, one day, be seen not only as 'complementary' to conventional medicine but as an essential part of a patient's overall healing process.

The stories and examples outlined in this book are taken from true life experiences. The recommendations I make are based on my own experiences, information supplied by qualified people and data obtained from reference books. Much of the information was also gained from listening and talking with the many people who passed through the doors of the Cancer Support Association.

If I were to be told that this book was simply a reflection of the representative view of

Chapter 1

the people who work with the various cancer organisations, then I would indeed be very pleased.

I am not a qualified nutritionist, nor a general practitioner or psychologist, but I did have cancer and have spent the past four years working as a carer, author and cancer/lifestyle speaker and therefore hope to relate to you, my reader, in an open and honest manner.

I stress that you should always seek appropriate guidance and advice before undertaking any formal or complementary course of treatment. Learn about the subject and then make your own decision and ensure that it is one with which you are completely comfortable and happy.

Accept your illness as a challenge, as a new beginning and an opportunity to look at life through 'new eyes'.

Happy reading.

CHAPTER 2

– A PERSONAL EXPERIENCE –

To any passer-by, the silhouette of two lonely figures standing embraced with heads lowered, in the middle of a nearly deserted hospital car park in Singapore, must have presented a sad and pathetic sight.

It was late December 1993 and my wife Katherine and I had just left the medical office of Dr Richard Chew, a leading Singaporean surgeon, after having our worst fears confirmed... I had been diagnosed with cancer; malignant melanoma which had metastasised (a lovely medical term meaning 'spread' into secondaries).

Twelve months earlier, my family and I had been posted from Perth, Western Australia to Singapore with my employment as marketing director for an Australian public company.

Although our life in Singapore was very stressful - with constant travel and playing host to a never ending stream of visitors - I had been generally in good health. The only exception was the onset of rheumatoid arthritis in my lower back. It had become progressively worse and my doctor had prescribed several drugs, which had not really helped.

A SMALL LUMP...

It was during mid-December 1993 whilst visiting Jakarta, Indonesia that I discovered a lump under my left arm. Although the lump was quite hard, it caused no pain, so I decided

Chapter 2

I should have it checked by my doctor back in Singapore as soon as possible.

Upon my arrival back in Singapore, 3 days later, I obviously didn't realise that our lives were about to change dramatically! Within two days I was diagnosed as having cancer in the form of a secondary malignant melanoma. Ironically, the primary melanoma could not be located, yet its 'offspring' had grown within my lymph glands, as a malignant tumor.

Whereas Singapore had excellent health facilities, they had not had a lot of experience with this type of cancer and it was therefore suggested that we return to live in Perth immediately. But the first thing I had to do was inform my family.

Once I had spoken to my parents and then to Katherine's parents (Alf and Beattie in Sydney), the remaining task of breaking the news to Jennifer and Gary (my Perth-based siblings) and to my brother Greg and sister-in-law Dominique (who live in France) was one of the most difficult undertakings of my life. Being close to my wife's family in Perth made my next task just as difficult!

By late January 1994 we were back in Perth and I had commenced combined chemotherapy and radiotherapy. The 'chemo' was to continue for 4 months and the radiotherapy for 5 weeks on a daily basis.

We had no home in Perth and all our belongings were in Singapore. Katherine had the enormous task of relocating our family and belongings, resettling the children into a new school and locating a home; not to mention finding time to visit her sick husband in hospital! It was only due to the support of our respective families that we got through this crisis.

My doctor advised me that melanoma tended to be 'very individualistic', with the prognosis that some patients would be 'OK' while other patients would deteriorate quite quickly. While he was reluctant to give a specific prognosis, he suggested my chances of a recovery were at best 'about 50-50'. Without 'chemo,' he advised, my chances were 'about 30%'.

With my whole life effectively 'turned upside down' I felt completely lost and devastated. My mind was confused and disoriented, yet I had to make a decision about the rest of my life, my values and future health... but, where to turn for help?

Chapter 2

During my hospital treatment I really didn't feel like doing anything and felt quite helpless and depressed, as the effects of the chemotherapy began to increase.

My cousin Lee told me about a group called The Cancer Support Association[1] and in March 1994, I reluctantly made my first visit, quite convinced that I would walk into a place full of sick cancer 'victims'. How wrong I was.

The C.S.A. was located in a lovely big old house called 'Wanslea' in Cottesloe (a western suburb about 15 minutes from the city of Perth) and was full of laughter and care.

It was here I was to learn about taking responsibility for my own recovery. Meditation, diet, physical fitness and a newly discovered spiritual awareness would, in conjunction with traditional medicines, create an environment which would give my body the very best chance to do what it wanted to do naturally... to heal!

Today, I meditate twice daily; drink 5-6 glasses of fresh vegetable juice every morning; eat fruit every day and consume primarily plant-based foods. I also swim 4 kilometres every week, at a local indoor pool.

I feel and look better than I have in many years. I have a blood pressure of 115:75 and enjoy perfect weight. I thank God for every day and enjoy my family and friends so much more. I also possess a wonderful sense of inner peace and calm.

And like so many cancer patients I had to examine my own background and acknowledge that to endlessly pursue the goal of saying 'yes' to everyone and wanting to be 'liked' by everyone was simply setting unrealistic targets which could never be achieved.

Today I still strive hard at my work and for various 'causes', but I have learned to not only pace myself and set achievable goals, but also to believe that I'm 'OK' and if that means not everyone is happy with Ross Taylor, well then, so be it!

And one final word... my arthritis has gone! Initially, my doctors explained that the chemotherapy would have reduced the effects of arthritis, however, after 4 years even they acknowledged that my lifestyle - and in particular diet - must have led to this amazing recovery from arthritis which is renowned for its debilitating effect on people.

CHAPTER 3

– WHAT CAN I DO TO HELP MYSELF? –

One of the worst feelings about being diagnosed with cancer is the complete sense of helplessness, anger and fear.

Questions thrash around the mind, seemingly out of control:

- Why me?
- Will I die soon?
- What about my family, my job?
- What are these treatments?
    - chemotherapy and radiotherapy
- Will I get even sicker?
- What can I do to help myself?
- Who can I turn to?
- How will my friends and employer react?

Doctors, and in particular oncologists, because of their type of work, generally believe that they cannot be in the 'hope' business. Accordingly they are often seen by cancer patients as cold, uncaring and most unsympathetic.

Chapter 3

This, combined with the apparent belief by many cancer specialists and doctors that there is nothing a cancer patient can do other than to present their diseased body for treatment, leads a patient to often experience extreme helplessness and fear.

Therefore, the first thing in dealing with cancer is to understand and believe that:

I CAN help myself to provide the best chance of recovery and to achieve an overall improvement in the quality of my life.

GETTING STARTED

For most people diagnosed with cancer, often a course of chemotherapy and radiotherapy would be recommended by your oncologist. It may also be recommended that the tumor be removed by means of surgery.

Some people will undertake the treatment, others will not, preferring a natural approach to healing. This is a decision you alone will have to make as there are arguments for and against.

Firstly, you should seek information and the various cancer organizations have some very good literature on this subject. They have offices throughout Australia and can be found in the local telephone directory.

The Cancer Foundation in Perth, Western Australia produces two small booklets entitled:

'CHEMOTHERAPY AND YOU'
and
'RADIOTHERAPY AND YOU'

Both books provide information that will be of assistance in understanding more about the treatment you are about to receive.

Chapter 3

Both the Cancer Support Association and the Cancer Foundation provide a wide range of information, books and tapes about cancer, and the various treatments. In the next chapter, I will briefly outline the likely types of treatment and the possible side effects.

Ironically for most people, it is quite common to find yourself 'hooked' up to a chemotherapy drip before you have even had time to decide if this is the course of treatment you wish to undertake!

YOUR RELATIONSHIP WITH YOUR ONCOLOGIST
(Cancer Specialist)

Once diagnosed with cancer, the relationship between doctor and patient becomes critical. A full understanding of the diagnosis, its implications and the procedures is obviously very important to every patient.

Yet sadly the vast majority of people with whom I have had contact found their doctors (oncologist) remote, unclear and confusing. Why should this be so?

My personal experience would support this view. Although my oncologist was highly regarded within his profession, both Katherine and I found our early meetings less than satisfactory.

It must be said, in fairness, that with so many thoughts 'thrashing' around your head it is not always easy to know exactly what to ask your doctor - or even comprehend what it is he or she is telling you.

After our first meeting, I thought I was to have 3 'lots' of chemo and 4 weeks of radiotherapy. In fact, I was to have 2x7 days of 'chemo' plus 35 consecutive days of radiotherapy, followed by a further regime of 'chemo' as an outpatient.

At this stage, I didn't understand that this would necessitate two full time residential stays in hospital for the chemo, yet the daily 'zap' of radiotherapy would take less than 30 seconds!

Chapter 3

WRITE IT DOWN

We quickly found that the best approach is to sit down before you visit the doctor and write out the questions that are on your mind or that you feel you need to ask. It is worth noting that the Cancer Foundation provides a helpful leaflet called 'Questions You Might Like To Ask Your Doctor' and this may assist you in preparing your questions.

At the surgery, tell your doctor that you have specific questions to ask and that you wish to write down the answers. Tell him it may take a little more time but that this is important to you. If you do not understand a reply ask for further explanation and clarification.

Another good alternative is to take a tape recorder along to each appointment. Your doctor should feel comfortable with this providing you explain what you intend to do.

DO NOT BE INTIMIDATED

Suffering from cancer often leaves people with low self esteem. It is common to walk into the oncologist's medical rooms feeling as though you are the poor diseased patient presenting your pathetic body to the doctor for assessment. Well, it need not be like that.

You have a disease for which you are now responsible. The doctor is there to serve you. He is being paid to provide the best professional assistance to you in your quest to becoming well again.

It is your absolute right to know exactly what the treatment will be, what options you have, what time and costs are involved and what you will be required to do.

So start by feeling good about yourself and you will quickly notice that your doctor will respond to you more effectively and openly!

If your relationship continues to be unsatisfactory it is your absolute right to seek out an alternative cancer specialist.

Chapter 3

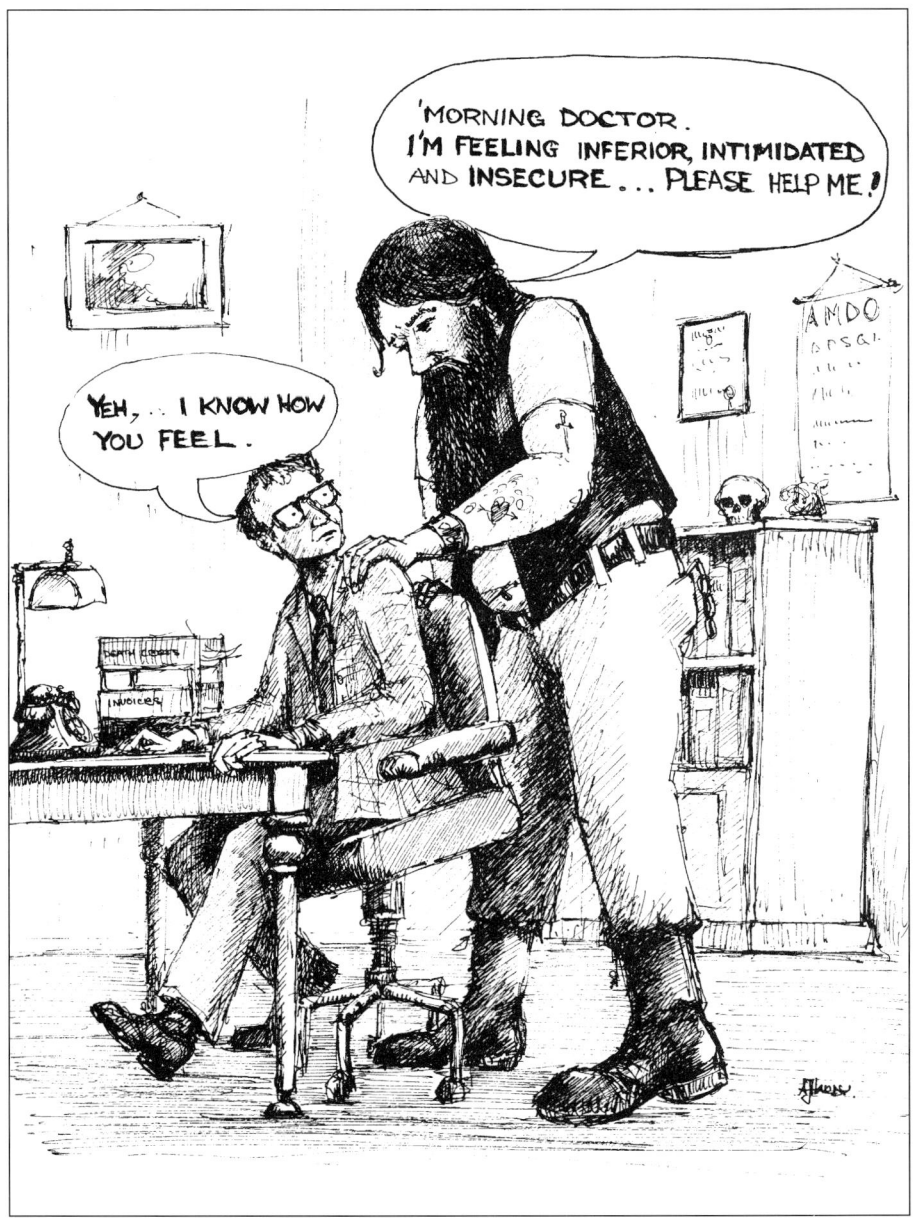

Chapter 3

DEVELOPING A 'TEAM' RELATIONSHIP WITH YOUR DOCTOR

It wasn't until I decided that the relationship with my oncologist HAD to change, that I actually set out to bring about these positive changes. This was achieved by putting myself on an equal 'one to one' basis rather than being just another submissive patient!

The actual method was, to say the least, quite unusual but most effective...

I noticed that each time I visited my oncologist, his secretary would always be the one to usher me into the surgery and that my doctor's desk was placed so that the patients would walk into the right and to the rear of his chair.

He would never stand or look up, preferring to mutter a vague 'morning' and point to the chair in front of the desk, whilst looking at his papers.

I decided this was unacceptable and that this habit represented my first challenge.

On the next visit, I was ushered in as usual by the secretary, however, this time I stopped just behind his chair and looked down over him.

'Good morning John*' I said, holding out my hand, whilst towering above him.

He reached up - from a totally submissive position to shake hands, responded 'err, um... good morning...'.

This was the greatest act of 'one upmanship' I had ever tried ... and it worked.

In future visits he would always enter the waiting room and invite me in personally and show me to my seat. Two months later, his desk was altered, so that he would actually face his patients as they entered the room. Within six months he actually relocated his entire office to new premises - although I can hardly claim responsibility for this move.

This was, however, a good starting point for improving our relationship.

(* A fictitious name)

Chapter 3

SOMEONE TO TALK WITH

As I explained earlier, cancer can often leave you frightened and very alone.

Not surprisingly, friends and family may also share the same feelings and often feel awkward in discussing the subject. Some people find that discussing a subject like cancer with loved ones is simply too emotional, and this only compounds the feelings of desperation and loneliness in everyone.

Help is available!

Most cities within Australia and overseas have groups that provide support for cancer patients and their families.

The Cancer Support Association in Perth and the Cancer Foundation has trained counsellors who can discuss with you, and your family if you wish the entire range of issues confronting you.

They can provide helpful advice concerning the complementary and alternative treatments available to you and how YOU can actually play a vital role in your own recovery. This initial counselling is of great importance in providing each patient with the information they need, upon which THEY can base their decisions about the pathway to be followed. In the end, it must be YOU who is comfortable and at peace with the treatments that you choose.

CANCER, STRESS AND THE IMMUNE SYSTEM

Evidence is now becoming available that supports the vital importance of people, when diagnosed with cancer, being able to access appropriate counselling and support groups.

In early 1998 Dr Barbara Andersen of the Ohio State University completed a research programme on 166 women, aged 31 to 84, who had recently been diagnosed with breast cancer.

Whilst it was known that cancer, in its own right, can significantly reduce the body's immune system, Dr Andersen's research showed that stress associated with the diagnosis of cancer ALSO contributed to the deterioration of the immune system.

Chapter 3

Adults who undergo chronic stress, such as the diagnosis and surgical treatment of breast cancer, often experience adjustment difficulties and important biologic effects, reports Dr Andersen.[2] The research highlighted the importance of helping patients deal with their cancer psychologically and physically.

Sadly, despite this new and mounting evidence, many cancer specialists simply diagnose their patient as having cancer and proceed to fight the disease through the use of drugs. No consideration is given to firstly looking at the causes of the cancer, and equally importantly, directing the patient to quality organisations which can provide support and a safe and caring environment whereby the patient can not only talk about their illness and how they feel, but also receive help as to how they can reduce stress (associated with the diagnosis of cancer) and improve their general health.

In my four years of working and being involved with cancer patients I have seen many examples where devastated and distraught people walk through the doors of the Cancer Support Association, seeking someone just to talk with. In many instances these people leave with a feeling of enormous relief at simply having had the opportunity to share their feelings and to learn that they are not alone or isolated.

A CASE IN POINT

Recently while participating in a television documentary about cancer, Channel 9's news presenter, Tina Altieri, was to introduce me (via a friend) to a young man who had been diagnosed with a brain tumor some nine months earlier. He was frustrated and distressed, saying that the doctors had said there was little that could be done with his form of cancer. Richard * understood this, but what he really needed was to be able to talk to other cancer patients and people who would listen to how he and his partner Gerda were really feeling.

Richard explained the following: 'We saw specialists in top hospitals in Holland and London before returning to Perth. At no time, despite our apparent distress, did anyone recommend counselling or support groups to us...'

*   All discussions at the support meetings are confidential unless authorised by the people concerned. Richard and Gerda gave approval for this story to be told for the benefit of others.

Chapter 3

They both decided to visit the regular support meetings which takes place every Tuesday and Thursday at the Cancer Support Association in Perth, Western Australia.

As they walked through the doors of this beautiful old building, the anxiety and heartbreak could be sensed. That first day, however, lead to incredible openness and 'letting go'.

During the following months Richard and Gerda discovered much about themselves, each other and the people around them. They have grown enormously, and while Richard must still deal with his brain tumor, he is now far more empowered and confident as a person to deal with this illness.

I sat and watched him playing his guitar (which he plays magnificently) for our group just before Christmas 1997 and reflected as he - and Gerda - joined the other cancer patients, carers and friends in laughter and song...

'Aah', I thought, 'how you both have grown in recent months.'

Both Richard and Gerda always had the ability to take control of this illness - all they needed was the initial support and the opportunity to simply talk with someone!

THE CARER – *A Most Difficult Task*

When someone is diagnosed with cancer, obviously the entire focus is on the patient. Yet, often the patient's carer (parent, spouse or close friend) will feel the impact just as much as the person diagnosed with cancer.

They are then faced with holding the whole family structure together, caring for the patient, seeking out the best treatments and answering a never-ending barrage of telephone calls and visitors' questions - all about the patient!

I asked my wife Katherine to express her feelings for inclusion in this book. Perhaps if you have been thrust into the carer's role you will relate to what Katherine has to say:-

'December 28th, 1993 is a day I will never forget. It is the day my whole world shattered into a million pieces, when I was informed that my soul-mate, best friend

Chapter 3

and husband of 16 years had secondary malignant melanoma. Ross was such an influential part of our lives and such a strong vibrant personality it was hard to accept that he had a life-threatening illness...

...As I had been a nurse who previously worked on the oncology ward plus some two years earlier my mother had cancer and passed away, this didn't leave me in a very positive frame of mind (about Ross' prognosis). The medical dictionary I read on secondary melanoma was soul-destroying.

I was in so much pain emotionally for everyone (Ross, myself and our two children)... Just to function on a day-to-day basis was extremely difficult. Ross' illness was constantly on my mind but I had to try very hard to be strong although I didn't always succeed - especially in Ross' company...

...During the treatment period in particular, all the attention is put on the person with the disease and meanwhile, the carer is going through so many emotions and just trying to come to terms with the whole situation as well as running a household and coping with the family...

...This is when close friends and family are important...

...We spoke openly about death and dying and the children were told the possible outcome. This was painful to do, but having experienced this very openly with my mother two years previously made it a little easier...

...I was already planning for the future. I bought a 'family' car as I would need this sized vehicle if Ross wasn't with us. I also had thought about what I would do with the house and was actively 'problem solving' before the 'problem' arose.

...I tried to get Ross to slow down; he did reduce his active life considerably but I felt he was still far too busy. I constantly 'nagged' him but he seemed to want to take his own course. It was then I realised that it was Ross who was - in the end - responsible for himself...

Chapter 3

Letting go can be very difficult, but realising and accepting that it was Ross who was in charge of his life and destiny - and that continually telling him to slow down was not going to work - finally allowed me to acknowledge that it is not the role of the carer to take the disease 'on board' themselves.

We did take a programme in Reiki (see Chapter 10) and Transcendental Meditation (T.M.) which jointly have changed our lives dramatically. I will always be grateful to Megan for introducing us to 'T.M.'...

...Reiki was also to be my saviour. I knew very little about it but intuitively knew I had to undertake the weekend course in Reiki for Ross' sake to help him relax and also for myself - an act of love which a lot of females rarely undertake...

...I have now learned to live for the moment, and appreciate the simple things in life. Today we both enjoy aromatherapy and relaxing music plus the new addition - a puppy called 'Penny' who has brought new joy into our lives...'

The emotions of loved-ones sometimes are all too similar. A friend of our family, Merrilyn saw life deal a cruel blow. She lost her first husband in a road accident; her second husband to lung cancer and her mother to bowel cancer.

To then learn that her son, Luke, had been diagnosed with Hodgkin's Disease (Lymphoma) should have been 'too much' for most people.

But through an incredible belief in herself and spirit, Merrilyn has survived. I asked her to reflect on her experience as a carer for her son...

'When my 21 year old son was diagnosed with Hodgkin's Disease I was deeply distressed; a normal reaction of most parents but I felt it was the end of the world, my worst nightmare realised. I was completely and utterly devastated.

When I was 22 years of age, with two sons and expecting my third child, my husband was killed in a traffic accident. At this time, my mother was suffering with terminal bowel cancer and died four weeks after my daughter was born, so it is little wonder the word 'cancer' invoked extreme apprehension.

Chapter 3

Looking back, I believe I became quite paranoid about death...

...Finally (thankfully) a wise clinic sister told me to 'live one day at a time' and I knew I had to do this if I wanted to stay sane...

...My son Luke turned 21 years of age on 31 October 1993...

...A few weeks prior to his birthday he showed me a lump on his neck...A lump is usually an indication of something amiss...

...On approximately 12 November, he mentioned 'the lump' appeared to be getting bigger. I was immediately concerned and advised him to see our doctor as soon as possible...

...On Wednesday, 17 November 1993, Luke was diagnosed with Hodgkin's Disease - a cancer of the lymphoid system...I was devastated to say the least - I think Luke was probably a little stunned by my reaction - I am ashamed to say I was unable to hide my feelings...

...My beloved son had cancer, one of my worst fears. I kept thinking 'why him? why not me' I could have handled it much better it if had been me. He was only 21, I was 42, I had had those extra years, his whole life was in front of him. The prospect of maybe losing one of my children, despite all the optimism, was unthinkable, but constantly with me. It was the most unbelievable nightmare. I also knew I had to pull myself together for his sake; he even said to me my reaction was 'bringing him down.'

...After my initial bad start in dealing with my son's illness, I realised that although this was a terrible thing to happen, I could not let it overwhelm me as it seemed to initially. I had a husband, three other children and a grandson, and if I was not careful I could shut them out. I did not want my fear of Luke's illness to take over my life as it could easily have done. As much for his sake as theirs. I had realised this from the beginning and apart from a couple of lapses, managed to do this. I am sure my husband and children were aware of how I felt within, but at least our lives were as normal as possible, given the circumstances...

...I think, as parents, we are inclined to blame ourselves for whatever goes wrong in

Chapter 3

our children's lives - whether it be some problem or even an illness, we feel ultimately responsible. We have failed! In those first dark days I wondered if maybe I was responsible for Luke having H.D., I thought perhaps it was diet related. Perhaps I hadn't provided the right foods and it had somehow lead to this! Quite bizarre really, because their diet was fairly healthy with plenty of vegetables, etc. Today I don't believe I caused him to contract this illness...

...It is almost five years since my son was diagnosed with Hodgkin's disease. He is extremely healthy and Dr x* is very optimistic...I owe him my son's life. But he is also a wonderful caring doctor, I would recommend him to anyone who is unfortunate enough to have cancer...

...I still don't like the word 'cancer' but it is no longer the death sentence it was. I now believe 'cancer is a word, not a sentence!'

If you are a carer, it is important to understand that it is 'normal' to feel cheated, angry, frustrated and often be left with a feeling of emptiness.

Counselling can often prove most beneficial and can help the carer to take control of their own lives and in doing so help the person for whom they care so much.

(*Doctor's original name has been removed for ethical reasons)

FEELING FOR THE FAMILY

I mentioned earlier that sometimes a patient may find it easier to seek outside counselling rather than talk it over with family members.

On occasions, this can leave some members of the family feeling hurt or thinking that they must have failed for you to turn for outside help. It is therefore helpful to always explain to loved ones that your sole objective is to get well again - which is obviously what they want for you.

By seeking external counselling and advice you are adding to the storehouse of knowledge that will allow you to make better and more relaxed decisions about what course of treatment and action you may take.

Conversely, sometimes relatives - particularly parents or a spouse - can become so busy

Chapter 3

running around seeking alternatives, looking for cures, and advising and planning, that they overlook the fact that perhaps the person they are so desperately trying to help may want them to slow down... and just listen to what they have to say.

The message, therefore, is simply: Be sensitive to each other and keep your communication lines - and minds - open!

MEN ARE NOT MOUNTAINS

I was perhaps not surprised to notice that the ratio of men diagnosed with cancer, who were seeking guidance, was dramatically lower than that of women.

I cannot specifically explain why but let me suggest that women tend to be far more 'in tune' with their bodies and 'aware' of their environment. They are often prepared 'to open up' and examine all the options and alternatives available before making any decision about their future and any course of treatment that they have been considering.

Men seem to have been taught to take a 'chin up' approach or adopt an attitude of 'don't worry it'll be OK'. One friend of mine solved his medical problem by heading off to the local pub and getting drunk!

Often underneath this strong tough-guy figure usually lies a soul that is just as confused and frightened as any woman and who desperately needs to talks things through and to seek counselling.

If you are a male, maybe now is a good time to 'let go'; get in touch with your feelings and teach yourself that it is 'okay' to open up and say how you feel and what it is that worries you most.

The first step is the most difficult, but after that you will experience a new feeling of calm and peace - and certainly a lot less stress!

Now is NOT the time to be deceiving yourself and others. So talk it over...

I cannot emphasise enough the importance of sitting down in a quiet and loving environment with an understanding carer, and simply talking about how you feel. The result can be amazing and can leave you with a sense of direction and a plan as to how you may progress from this point.

CHAPTER 4

– CONVENTIONAL TREATMENTS –

Just the mention of chemotherapy and radiotherapy can create fear amongst many patients, so it is therefore worthwhile for me to discuss both forms of treatment (albeit briefly) which often will occur alongside other forms of treatment such as surgery.

CHEMOTHERAPY

The name chemotherapy is believed to have originated from the words 'chemicals' and 'treatment'. Hardly a combination that generates excitement, but for many people 'chemo' does play an important role in their overall treatment. The primary function of chemotherapy is to seek out cancer cells (fast growing ones) and destroy them before they begin to multiply.

Chemotherapy is administered usually by means of an intravenous drip over a short or long period. It can also be administered by means of a catheter, orally, or sometimes by injection. It is seldom painful.

Your doctor should carefully plan the course of chemotherapy to be given and, as previously indicated, you should discuss details of the programme with him or her thoroughly before starting, as each particular regime can differ significantly. While some patients I knew would receive a one-hour intravenous dose each day, I received 2 lots of 7 days (24 hours per day) administered as an in-patient at a hospital.

Chapter 4

Types of Chemotherapy

Chemotherapy treatment can consist of one or a combination of drugs.

Side Effects of Chemotherapy

There can be a number of side effects resulting from chemotherapy.

As the aim of 'chemo' is to destroy the fast growing cancer cells it is possible for the drugs to also attack other fast growing cells. These may include:

- Cells within the mouth resulting in mouth ulcers.
- Cells within the throat resulting in sore or burning throat.
- Cells for producing hair resulting in partial or complete hair loss.
- Cells that may affect hearing.
- Bone marrow cells which can be seen in the form of bruising or anaemia.
- White cells resulting in lowered immune system (low blood count).

It should be noted that many patients - myself included - did not experience any significant side effects; some were affected by only one or two of the above, whilst others would become quite sick on the first day of treatment.

Probably, the most common side-effect is that of nausea, which can occur either on day 1 or not until well into the treatment.

Fortunately, our bodies can recover and replace any damaged cells within a relatively short period... and yes, your hair will grow back!

Diet

Often during chemotherapy treatment you may find your mouth becoming dry and sore and the desire for food diminished.

It is important during and after treatment, that you absorb as much wholesome fresh food

Chapter 4

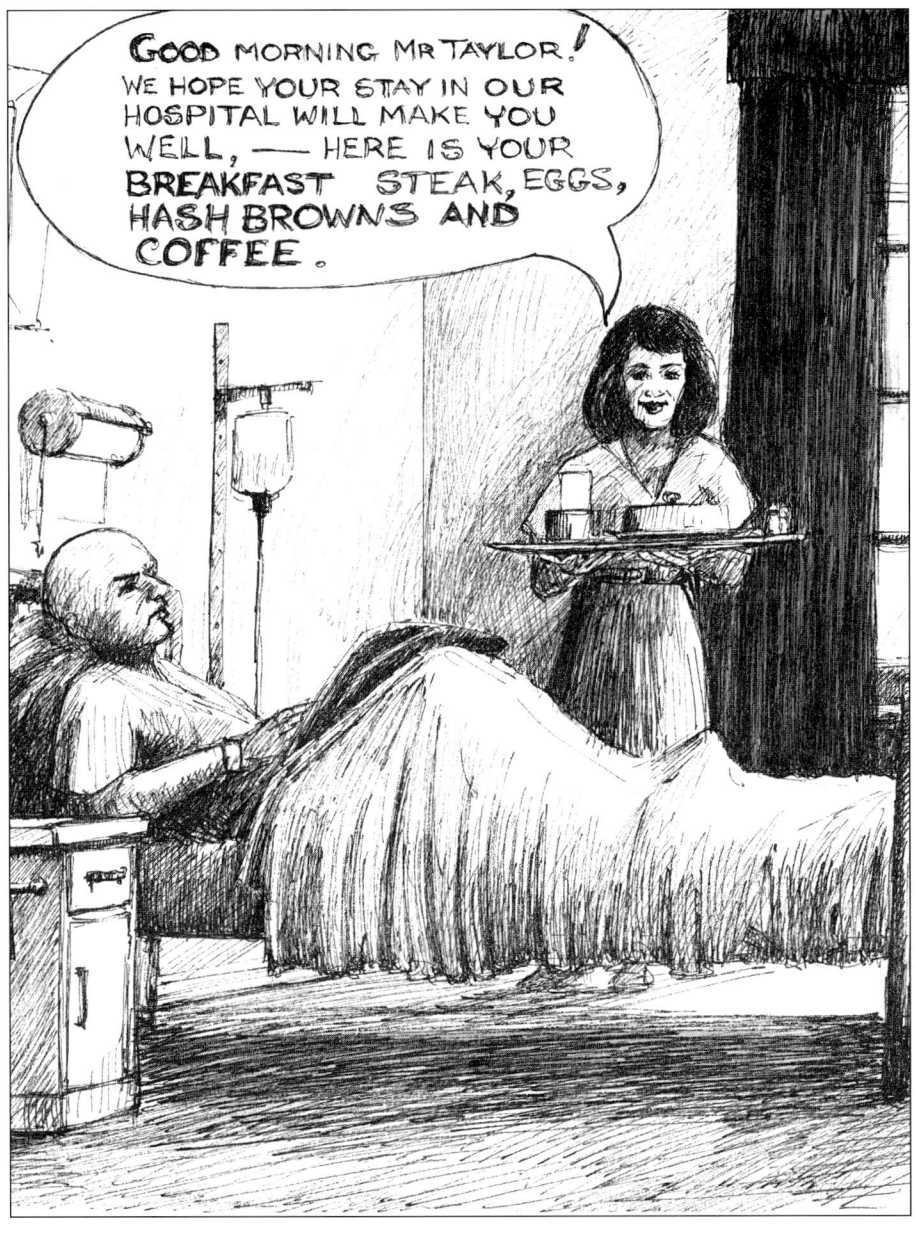

Chapter 4

as possible. I can remember my first day in hospital being offered a meal of instant chicken soup, hot roast beef roll and apple pie and ice cream ... and they were supposed to be preparing my body for the onset of chemotherapy drugs!

In the following chapters, I will discuss the important issue of diet in considerable detail, but if on one given day you just can't cope with consuming food, don't be overly concerned; try again the next morning as your appetite can change quite quickly.

RADIOTHERAPY

Whilst chemotherapy is designed to 'flow' through the entire body, radiotherapy is localised.

Radiotherapy is used specifically at a particular area - often at the site of a tumor or from where a tumor has been removed.

The most common form of radiotherapy is 'external radiotherapy' which is radiation administered under strict guidelines and by highly skilled staff.

The Treatment

During your initial visit, the staff will probably take normal X-Rays of the affected area. They will then have you lie on a bed under the simulator, while they 'mark' your skin. This is a painless but important function to plan the precise area to receive the radiotherapy. In this way, all non-affected areas can be shielded from the radiotherapy rays.

Depending on the type of cancer, the treatment may take place once or twice daily for a period usually of between 4 - 7 weeks.

Each particular treatment lasts only a few minutes - the longest part being the wait for your turn in the seemingly always busy clinics!

There is no pain associated with radiotherapy. In fact, you cannot feel anything, with the side effects only noticeable after a number of treatment sessions.

Chapter 4

Side Effects

The possible side effects of radiotherapy are similar to those for chemotherapy (see previous pages), however, are often localised to the particular area being treated.

The only noticeable side effect I experienced was the skin rash that developed by the third week. The skin took on the appearance of someone with a bad rash or sunburn. The doctor can recommend creams to place on the affected area.

If you live near a beach and your treatment is during the summertime, your skin will respond very positively to a 'dip' in the ocean. Remember, however, the skin can become very sensitive to the sun during radiotherapy so it is therefore essential to bathe in the early morning or late afternoon.

Relations with Family and Friends

During 'chemo' and radiotherapy your body is undergoing a rigorous 'assault' as the drugs attempt to attack and destroy the cancer cells, so it is not unusual to come home from hospital feeling tired and often very 'touchy' or sensitive.

Take time to explain to your loved ones that this is a difficult time for you and ask for their support - even if you are grumpy!

The Decision To Undertake Chemotherapy and Radiotherapy

This is a decision you will make yourself after considering all the information available to you. As I have indicated, I did choose to have both chemotherapy and radiotherapy because I saw the treatments as complementary to my body's natural desire to heal itself.

I often agonized, however, over what exactly to say to cancer patients about chemotherapy - as for many people (including myself in those early days) 'chemo' represents their major hope in fighting cancer, and particularly when the cancer specialists support its use. After time, however, you will learn that in some cases chemotherapy can assist but see it as part of an overall 'package' involving conventional and complementary programmes.

Whilst chemo does have success with some cancers - such as childhood leukemia - it must be said that it has not lived-up to the high expectations it promised when first discovered just after the Second World War.

It is true that 'chemo' does attack cancer cells but unfortunately it also attacks other fast growing cells (hair, eyes, hearing) often turning the body into something of a battleground.

Sometimes doctors will refer to successful chemotherapy 'response rates'. I, like many cancer patients, believe this means 'cure rates' when in reality it means that the tumor may have responded positively to the treatment usually without consideration to the possibility of the tumor re-appearing somewhere else.

Yet at the same time one cannot help but wonder at the true marvel of the human body. This amazing gift called life can not only develop its own intelligence but can automatically self-correct and heal itself. This should always be considered when deciding on whether to proceed with treatments such as chemotherapy.

This is not to say you should be frightened off by chemotherapy - but you should have a clear understanding about this drug; its side effects and the actual success rate with your type of cancer.

Your attitude to these treatments is vitally important. If you undertake chemotherapy because you see it as helping you to achieve a full recovery, then that is fine. Alternatively, if you undertake the treatment because 'I'll die if I don't' then perhaps you need to seek some counselling to ensure you approach your treatment with a positive attitude, or if there is not an alternative approach that you are actually seeking.

Further Information

Contact the Cancer Foundation or ask your doctor for literature on the various forms of cancer treatment. The more you read and understand about what is happening to you, the more you will be able to prepare for the task ahead.

CHAPTER 5

– CREATING THE HEALING ENVIRONMENT –

Whilst it is always dangerous to generalise, of the many people I have met who have been diagnosed with cancer, they inevitably fall into one of three categories. (Note that it is quite common for some people to move 'in and out' of the following three scenarios.)

The first category has the following 'mind-set' and outlook:

> 'Just my luck that I'd get cancer'
> 'Everything bad happens to me'
> 'Not much I can do - doctor says the only thing is chemo'
> 'Self help? Nah, no point...'

The second group are gripped by denial:

> 'I just don't want to know about this'
> 'We don't discuss matters like cancer'
> 'My husband doesn't like to talk'
> 'I can't even think about what's happening to me, let alone talk about it'
> 'Just pretend that it isn't happening'

The third group adopts a 'mind-set' which is something like this:

> 'Sure I was devastated, but I'm confident that I can recover'

Chapter 5

'If my body created this cancer, then surely my body can also heal itself'

'There are many things I can do to improve my quality of life and overall prognosis'.

This is not said lightly for if you REALLY wish to do something about your diagnosis, you must be genuinely prepared to make some changes. The extent of changes will be up to you, but the objective should be to create an environment whereby your body has the best opportunity to heal itself.

FOUR KEY AREAS

During my days in hospital attached to the 'chemo' drip, I had the opportunity to reflect on this matter carefully. After much reading of both Western and Eastern treatment options plus counselling and careful consideration, I finally decided that there were four main areas where I needed to focus my attention, and I would like to discuss these with you now:-

i)	*The inner body functions*	*(diet)*
ii)	*The power of the mind*	*(meditation)*
iii)	*The outer body*	*(physical fitness)*
iv)	*Spiritual*	*(me and my God)*

I came to the conclusion that if I could get these four areas 'in harmony', my body would be given a correct environment for it to undertake the natural task of healing.

Once I accepted this philosophy, the task ahead did not seem such a major challenge after all and in fact almost became exciting!

I need to stress, right now, the absolute importance of defining your own set of goals or your own programme.

The four 'key' areas which we will look at in the coming chapters have proven most successful FOR ME. Other cancer survivors have defined areas for which they give priority. I know, without doubt, that my wife Katherine would have 'Reiki' listed in the first two

Chapter 5

priority items... this is fine... so long as you are completely happy that the programme you have chosen is something to which you can give your total commitment, and with which you feel completely at ease.

Over the next four chapters, I will examine my own experiences - and make suggestions - regarding these key areas affecting the whole human being.

CHAPTER 6

– DIET –

(INNER BODY FUNCTIONS)

A number of oncologists hold the view - and sadly convince their patients - that a change in diet will do nothing to assist in their patients' recovery or improve their quality of life.

Evidence is mounting, however, that in fact dietary changes can certainly assist greatly during chemo and radiotherapy and also have a direct effect on the overall improvement in the short and long term health of a patient.

Initially, I must admit I was somewhat sceptical about this 'wholesome fresh food' concept, until I spoke to a bio-chemist in mid 1994.

He asked if I had noticed that during summer in Perth, many of the palm trees turn yellow. Having worked in the agriculture business, I could relate to this and understood that yellow leaves is often a result of a lack of the essential elements such as potassium and magnesium.

He went on *'...imagine if you were to reduce the amount of water (fluids) and also put half a bag of salt on your palm trees each month; increase the acid in the soil rather than the alkalinity; and withdraw the dose of nutrients that you had been applying regularly... you probably wouldn't be surprised if your palm looked lifeless, became 'sick' and eventually died.'*

Chapter 6

Yet in many aspects, this is exactly what we do to our own bodies.

In fact, many of us even add an additional dose of nicotine. It is indeed a miracle that despite this massive assault on our bodies through poor diet, we continue to live at all!

WHAT FOODS ARE BEST

In my search for answers, I discovered that a good diet is not only about fat and cholesterol - that we hear so much about. It is also about getting the body chemically balanced. It sounds complicated but actually it is all quite simple and makes good logical sense.

In determining an appropriate diet for healing we should aim to consume foods that are 80% alkaline-based and foods that are 20% acid-based, as this is the requirement our body demands, in order to perform efficiently.

Any significant variation to this, leaves the body chemically 'imbalanced', and operating less efficiently.

Unfortunately for many people in Western countries, our diet is almost the opposite (ie) 80% acid and 20% alkaline ... and yet, we act surprised when we become ill! Let's look at alkaline and acid foods:

Alkaline Forming Foods (80%)

Alfafa	Carrots	Parsley
Almonds	Cucumber	Parsnip
Apples	Currants	Paw paw
Apricots	Dates	Peaches
Artichoke	Eggplant	Pears
Asparagus	Garlic	Persimmons
Avocado	Goats Milk - Fresh	Potato Peels
Bananas	Grape Juice	Prunes
Beans - Kidney	Grapes	Pumpkin
Beans - String	Honey - Unrefined	Radish
Beetroot	Horseradish	Raisins
Broccoli	Juice - Vegetable	Snow Peas

Chapter 6

Broth - Vegetable	Kale	Sorrel
Cabbage - Red	Kelp	Soya Beans
Cabbage - White	Kohirabi	Spinach
Capsicum	Leek	Sprouts
Cauliflower	Lettuce - Cos	Squash
Celery	Mushrooms	Sultanas
Cherries	Ochra	Swiss Chard
Chicory	Olives - Black	Tomatoes - very ripe
Coconut	Olive Oil - cold press	Water Cress
Cantaloupe	Onions	Zucchini

Acid Forming Foods (20%)

Bacon	Fish*	Potatoes
Barley	Flour - Gluten	Rabbit
Beans	Flour - Rye	Rice - Brown
Beef	Flour - Wheat	Rice - Flour
Bread - Rye	Goose	Rice - Noodles
Bread - Wholemeal	Grapefruit	Rice - White
Butter	Ham	Ricecakes
Buttermilk	Ice cream	Ricotta Cheese
Carob	Jelly	Sausages
Cashew nuts	Lamb	Shellfish
Cereals - Oats, Bran	Maize*	Soya Cheese
Chestnuts	Milk - nonfat	Soya Pasta
Chicken	Millet	Spaghetti Wholemeal
Chocolate	Mutton	Sugar - Raw
Cocoa	Nuts	Sugar - White
Corn	Oatmeal*	Takeaway foods
Corn meal	Pasta - wheatfree*	Tapioca
Corn starch	Peanuts	Turkey
Cottage Cheese	Peas - dried	Turtle

Living Simply With Cancer

Crackers	Pecan nuts	Veal
Dairy Products	Pies & Pastries	Vinegar - Apple Cider
Duck	Pork	Yoghurt - Kefir
Eggs		

* Only slightly acid forming (almost neutral)

So, try and choose foods that will provide you with the 80:20 ratio. It doesn't mean you can't enjoy some acid or neutral foods (bread, potatoes and pasta provide an excellent source of fibre and carbohydrate); just seek out an appropriate balance.

POTASSIUM AND SODIUM

Potassium is an essential element, that acts in many ways to improve cell structure, assists the kidneys to detoxify blood and maintains the alkaline/acid ratio in the blood and body tissues.

The ratio of potassium/sodium is now generating great interest. As early as 1920 a German physician, Dr Max Gerson[3], was claiming that many chronic illnesses could be related back to an imbalance between potassium and sodium.

We should, according to Gerson, have a potassium to sodium intake of about 4:1.

His theory was that potassium rich foods would generate and activate the white cells within the body - these are the cells that attack and destroy cancer and other illness related cells.

Being interested by Gerson's work and conclusions, I decided to seek out other expert views. Through my friend in Singapore, Robert Yam, I was to contact Dr Lai Chiu-Nan, who now resides in America, but is still highly recognised within Asia for her research and knowledge about cancer and its treatment. Dr Lai holds a PhD in chemistry and has written a book, 'The Pursuit of Life'[4]. I was fascinated with what Dr Lai had to say about potassium and sodium:

'Let me emphasise the importance of the potassium/sodium ratio. In our research it was found that increasing the potassium level in the growth media can revert cancer cells to normal cells. The best potassium source in food is vegetables. The high potassium foods are vegetables and fruits. The poor potassium sources are animal or processed food.'

Dr Lai went on to say:

'For cells to perform normally, they need to concentrate potassium and expel sodium. In the cells, potassium to sodium ratio is about 10 times. When cell membranes are damaged, potassium is leaked and the cells start to divide. Dividing cells and cancer cells have a lower ratio of potassium to sodium compared to normal cells. That cancer cells grow in an uncontrolled manner is probably related to the lowered potassium-sodium ratio...

...Why am I emphasising the ratio of potassium and sodium in food? Because it plays a role not only in cancer but also in high blood pressure, heart diseases, and diabetes.'

Dr Lai also found during her research, that in the U.S. the average intake of potassium over sodium is about 0.7; less than the body constitution, which is around 2:1. Cancer, heart diseases and diabetes are common in the U.S., and can be attributed to this factor in the diet. Chinese in general eat more rice and vegetables, and it appears their risk of getting these diseases is less.

If you think your family regularly has a food balance of 4:1 of potassium over sodium, just read the ingredients section on almost any packaged food (including cereals) in your pantry, but this time don't just look for cholesterol and fat content, but examine the ratio between potassium and sodium. The findings will shock you.

In fact, one of the world's leading brands of corn flakes boasts a ratio of 29mg potassium to 280mg sodium for every serve!

WHAT SORT OF FOODS TO CONSUME

Easily Digestible Foods

Foods that take a long period to be digested have a far greater opportunity of fermenting and putrefying within the body, thus creating toxins around the blood stream.

Fat Free or Fat Reduced Foods

Obviously foods that are free of cholesterol and saturated fat are preferable.

Chapter 6

Fresh Vs Organic

While organically grown food is highly desirable, it may not always be possible to obtain produce which is organic. Therefore aim to obtain freshly picked/grown foods whenever possible. Scrub vegetables before eating or juicing.

I am becoming increasingly concerned, however, that so many of our raw foods are 'bathed' in chemicals and insecticides to kill off insects. But what is it doing to us humans?

DAIRY FOODS

I am sure there was no one who enjoyed dairy foods - and in particular milk - more than me. A 10pm snack of corn flakes flooded with fresh cold milk... mmm! Today, I would never even consider drinking a glass of dairy milk.

When Louis Pasteur invented the method of pasteurizing milk, the world was given a product that would last longer and be mostly disease free. We would also get a product that was effectively 'cooked', hence destroying the living enzymes and also the friendly bacteria, which is essential in protecting the body.

In the process of cooking, the proteins are changed into a denser form of curd which are three times the levels of human (mother's) milk. This makes the product extremely hard to digest. In fact when cows' milk reaches the stomach the curd 'wraps' around other food, insulating and inhibiting its digestion until the curd itself is completely broken down.

'But you need milk for calcium and to prevent osteoporosis', I hear you say.

In America today there are some 18 million victims of osteoporosis, yet America has amongst the highest intake of cows' milk in the world. England, Sweden and Finland also have amongst the highest consumption of milk - and also have amongst the highest levels of osteoporosis - in the world! Yet in many African and Asian countries which have low or no dairy milk intake there is a much lower level of bone disease. In some cases osteoporosis is unheard of.[5] In fact evidence is mounting that a person on a diet which is excessively high in protein may actually experience an increase in the amount of calcium lost from their bones.

Since I stopped consuming dairy milk, the years of allergies, 'runny nose' and sinus have suddenly stopped.

Rice or soy milk are excellent substitutes. There are a number of excellent soy-milk products now available such as the organically-grown 'Bonsoy' (my 13 year-old daughter even likes it!) and also 'Vita-Soy', which is a great tasting organically grown product.

A CHOICE TO MAKE

The most difficult task I faced was to make a choice of those products I would eliminate completely from my future diet, those products I would only consume in small quantities, and those foods I would substantially increase in my overall intake.

i) *Eliminate Completely*

Tea & Coffee	(replace with herbal teas)
Dairy products	(replace with soy products)
All red meats	(beef; lamb; pork; mutton etc)
Confectionery	(try dates and almonds - they are great!)
Desserts & Puddings	(fruit salads taste better)
Mayonnaise, Margarine & Butter	(if you must have something on your bread, try cold pressed virgin olive oil, or in a sandwich, use fresh avocado as a spread)
Sugar	(including brown sugar)
All take-away foods	(especially fried foods)
Soft drinks	(juice up your own fruits)
Ice cream products	(well, once in a while if you really have to!)

I have deliberately omitted alcohol from this list for two reasons.

Chapter 6

The first is that there is now sufficient evidence to suggest one glass of red wine per day can be of benefit (the crushed grape seed is one of the most powerful anti-oxidants known).

Secondly, I can think of nothing better than on a spring day to sit with friends over a pasta and salad lunch whilst sipping on a glass (just one glass!) of Australian shiraz.

MY ANNUAL ICE CREAM TREAT

Each year my family and I travel 3 hours south of Perth, to the beautiful wine growing region of Margaret River. It is at the nearby town of Dunsborough one can find what I firmly believe is the best ice cream in the world!

Simmo's Ice Creamery is operated by a young man called Garth (who incidentally I have never formerly met) and the range and quality of ice cream is truly mind boggling. Now let me not confuse you; ice cream is definitely something that cancer patients should not be eating on a regular basis, however, for a once a year treat this simply can't be beaten.

In fact I even have a friend in England who swears he would gladly make the trip from London to Dunsborough just to eat a Simmo's Ice Cream!

The issue here is an important one… if your diet is so rigorous and strict that your life becomes a misery, then what is the point? For me a glass of wine with friends over a good meal, and my once a year ice cream from Simmo's IS living, and that is what really matters!

So ensure your diet is 'livable' and an enjoyable experience.

ii) *Consume In Limited Quantities*

    Free range chicken *   (but remove the skin first)

    Fish *   (deep sea varieties)

    Soy based ice cream   (only very occasionally as it does contain preservatives etc.)

*   It should be noted that since preparing this book I have now reduced my intake of chicken to only once a week. This makes me an (almost) vegetarian!

Chapter 6

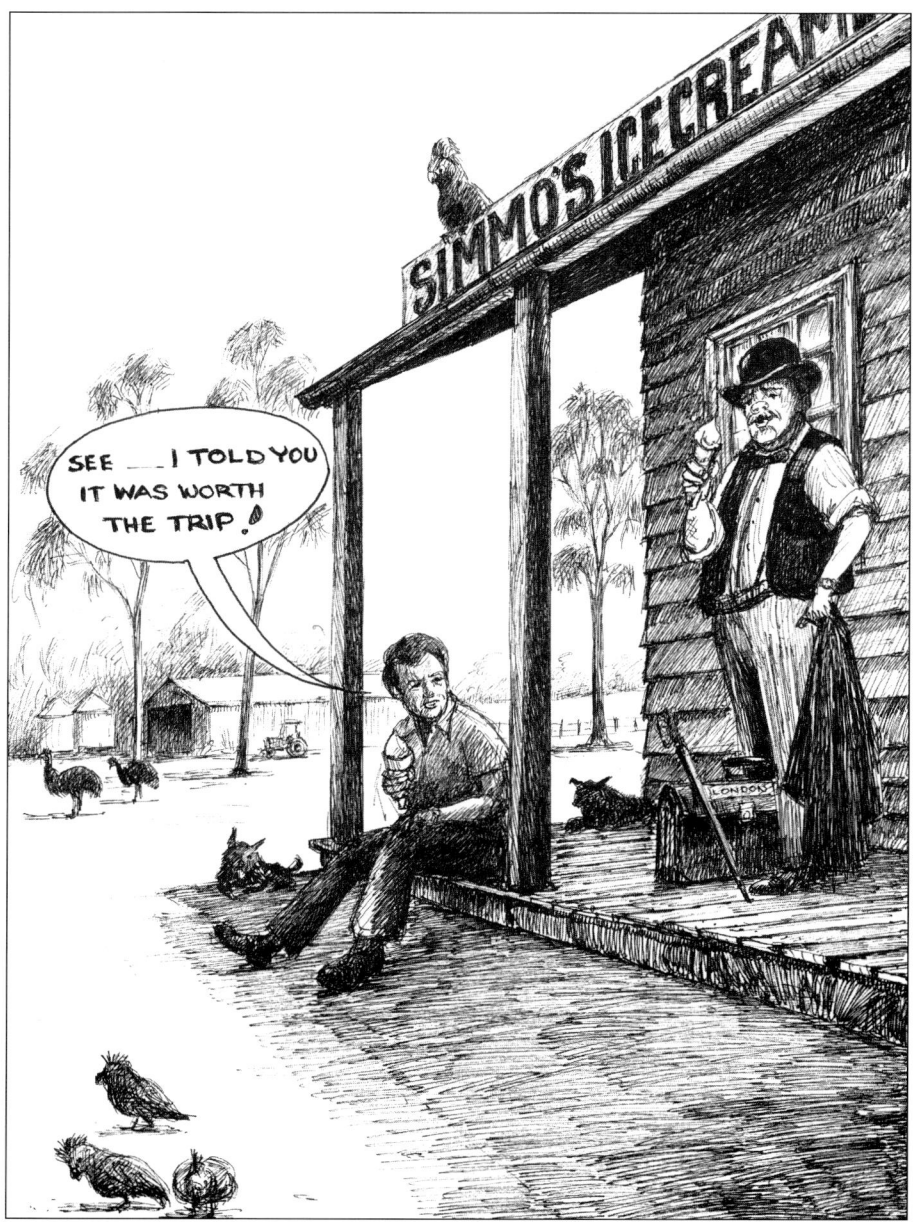

Chapter 6

	Eggs	(perhaps in the form of egg-based pasta rather than as fried or boiled eggs)

iii) *Increase Intake Significantly of:*

Fresh vegetables	
Fresh fruits	
Raw vegetable and fruit juices	(See separate section on juices)
Nuts	(Almonds only)
Whole grains	(Brown rice, lentils, oat or maize porridge, pasta and breads)

While one's first reaction may be 'oh there's no way I can follow this diet', it really is quite simple - and remember, you will quickly feel so much better.

A SPECIAL LOOK AT JUICING

It is a medically nutritional fact that a constant supply of high quality nutrients in the correct quantities and blends will inevitably result in a human body that becomes healthy, alive and functions efficiently.

In June 1993, an article written by Gladys Block[6] in the Journal of the National Cancer Institute stated that 'there can be no disagreement that people should eat a balanced diet rich in fruit, vegetables and whole grains... The antioxidants (of these foods) have a definite role of reducing the risk of some cancers'.

In Julie Stafford's excellent book 'Juicing for Health'[7], we can quickly see the enormous benefits gained from juicing fresh vegetables and fruits. Julie goes on to say:

- 'Juices are full of nutrients and enzymes that help fight diseases and promote a healthy and strong immune system

- Juices provide instant nutrition and because they are fibre free, are rapidly absorbed into the blood stream and go to work immediately - healing, energising, revitalising and generating healthy growth

Chapter 6

- Juices provide instant sustainable energy
- Juices can assist by alleviating stress by correcting the body's acid/alkaline balance (see earlier pages), and
- Juices are filling and while being low in kilojoules and high in water, they also speed up the body's metabolism.'

If you do nothing else but add fresh juices to your diet, you will feel and look better within a short time and enjoy new found energy.

Since starting to enjoy natural freshly juiced vegetables and fruit, I have planned my daily routine to ensure I always have access to these wonderful drinks.

TRAINING HOTEL STAFF

In my business life, I have to travel regularly overseas to South-East Asia, yet within the space of only 12 months I have 'trained' hotel staff in Jakarta, Singapore, Kuala Lumpur and Bangkok to cater for my desire to consume fresh juices.

One particularly helpful young lady (named Rena) at Singapore's Pan Pacific Hotel is so well tuned-in to my drinking habits, she inevitably rings my hotel room telephone before I have even unpacked my bags after arrival...

'Good evening Mr Taylor; welcome back to the Pan Pacific Hotel; would you like your carrot and celery juice now...'

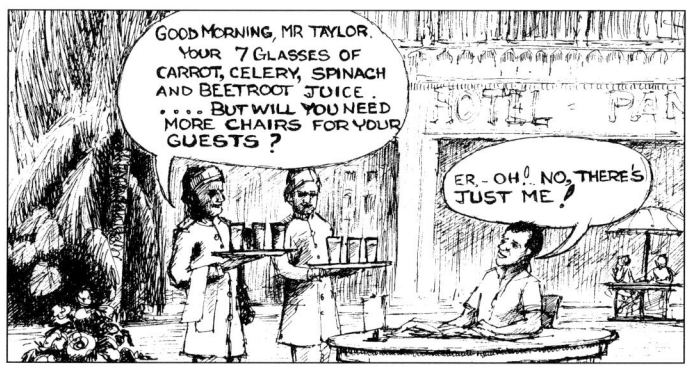

Chapter 6

Even around the hotel pool (on the rare occasions I get to enjoy the facility), I only have to raise my hand and the poolside steward is there.

'Ah Mr Taylor... would you like a vegetable juice!!'

During chemotherapy and/or radiotherapy you may feel you cannot even look at a glass of juice (or any other food for that matter) let-alone actually consume it! In fact, even just one or two daily glasses of fresh juice will help offset the effects on your system caused by 'chemo' and radiotherapy.

IS BOTTLED JUICE OK?

Within hours of being bottled, most juices will have lost many of the vitamins and minerals essential to the body.

Do yourself a favour, take the time to make up your own juice - fresh each day, and drink it all within 30 minutes of juicing to ensure you gain maximum benefit. It also will taste so much better, and those horrible 'free radicals' will not have had the time to oxidise and destroy the living enzymes from the juice.

WHEN TO ENJOY FRESH JUICES

Juices can be enjoyed at any time, but I personally have found that first thing in the morning is the best time to enjoy vegetable juice. They certainly 'fill you up', leaving you quite happy until lunch time, or at least mid morning.

There is another important reason to enjoy fresh juice first thing in the morning on an empty stomach. Under these circumstances the vegetable juice is fully digested within 15-20 minutes from the time it is consumed. The body is able to use this 'living food' immediately to nourish and replenish the tissues, cells and glands - with almost no effort on the part of the digestive system.

In addition these wonderful juices assist greatly in re-oxygenating the blood - this vital oxygen which is almost entirely lost when food is cooked.

Upon arriving home from work or in the late afternoon (preferably around 2-3 hours after the last food intake) enjoy one or more fruit-based juices. It is also cheaper than drinking

Chapter 6

2 or 3 stubbies of beer or a 'scotch and coke'.

WHAT JUICES ARE BEST?

For people being treated for, or recovering from, cancer here is my own personal choice - although there are many different varieties and blends available. There are also a number of excellent books available at good book shops, with recipes for fruit and vegetables that can be easily juiced.

Vegetable Juicing

Carrots

Carrots are probably the most common and versatile of all vegetables used for juicing.

Carrot juice is high in:

Vitamin A (beta carotene)	Potassium
Calcium	Magnesium

Carrots give excellent flavour and appearance to any juice and provide a good base for blending, with other vegetables.

Celery

Celery is high in organic sodium (the 'OK' type of sodium); potassium; phosphorous and blends well with carrots.

Parsley

Parsley is a herb, not a vegetable, but as a member of the 'green' family, it is a great cleanser. Parsley should be taken in only small quantities. (One small handful is usually quite sufficient).

Beetroot

A wonderful 'blood builder' that combines well with other juices. In addition to being rich in iron, beetroot also contains 9 essential minerals and 4 of the major vitamins. Beetroot is very 'earthy' in taste so it is best used in small to medium quantities.

Chapter 6

Spinach

I prefer what we, here in Australia, call 'English Spinach'. It tastes great as a salad and even better as a juice. It is quite sweet in taste and blends well with other juices.

As one of the 'green' foods, spinach is a great blood cleanser.

Spinach is also rich in vitamins A, B & C, plus calcium, magnesium, phosphorous and potassium: it really is a marvellous food. Remember, however, that spinach does contain oxalic acid so it is probably best to consume in small to medium quantities only, if you suffer any aches or joint pains, and wish to cook this food.

Lettuce

For some reason, I always believed lettuce was a nutritionally devoid food. I was very wrong!

Easy to juice, lettuce is a good source of calcium, chlorophyll and potassium. It also contains vitamins A & E and is also a good blood cleanser.

There are many other wonderful vegetables, including cucumber, parsnip and the marvellous broccoli, which is somewhat more difficult to juice, but can be introduced to your juicing programme.

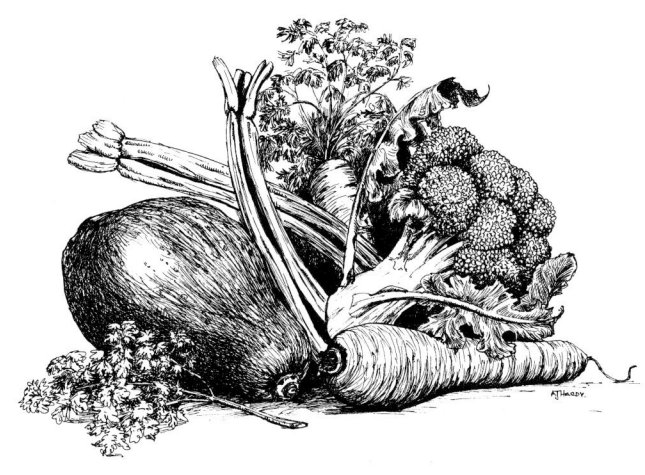

Chapter 6

HOW TO MAKE FRESH JUICES
WHAT COMBINATIONS AND QUANTITIES SHOULD I USE?

It is generally accepted that the body requires 8-10 glasses of liquid per day. Instead of drinking coffee, tea, beer and soft drink, switch to vegetable and fruit juices - and feel the difference.

The quantity and combinations is really up to you, but personally I drink around 5 glasses of fresh vegetable juice every morning as soon as I rise from bed, and 1-2 glasses of fruit juice late in the day. During the middle of the day try and drink 2-3 glasses of purified water, or some herbal teas which are now readily available at most shops, cafes, and hospital cafeterias.

I have developed a particular juice blend that is 'OK' with my system. You may like to try this. The following 'recipe' will provide 5-6 glasses so reduce the quantities listed according to your desired intake - remember it may be better to start with smaller quantities and increase the intake progressively.

- 6 - 8 medium size carrots
- 3 sticks celery
- 2 slices beetroot
- 1 handful lettuce
- 1 small handful parsley
- 1 handful English spinach
- 1 apple

(It is probably not a good idea to mix fruit and vegetables - enjoy them separately. The only exception is the apple which adds a sweet taste to vegetable juice and chemically and nutritionally blends well with vegetables.)

Prior to juicing, scrub the carrots (rather than peeling) and thoroughly wash the other vegetables, and ... do yourself a favour, buy a good quality juicer as it will save you a lot of time and frustration. Champion Juicers are excellent and I recommend them.

Chapter 6

Once you have juiced the 6 vegetables and 1 apple, drink the juice progressively over the next 30-45 minutes and enjoy. Even swirl the liquid around in your mouth before swallowing, allowing the nutrients to enter through the pores of your skin.

As a pleasant variation, I often add a few pieces of broccoli, capsicum and 3-4 slices of cucumber. The taste becomes a little more bitter but quite refreshing to the palate.

You can also experiment by adjusting the overall quantities to taste or adding varieties of other vegetables such as parsnip or watercress if you wish.

Five to six glasses of this juice will leave you hunger free until lunch time - and for the first time, perhaps, you will even sense your body telling you how good it feels, leaving you wondering how you could have ever believed the myth about the need for a big hearty breakfast every morning 'to get you started'.

About the only thing a big hearty breakfast of steak and eggs will do is send you running to the coffee-maker to stop your body from going to sleep!

A BODY CLEANSING PROGRAMME

It is unfortunate that as our lives become more stressful and the pace of life increases, the concept of enjoying food at a leisurely pace has almost become a thing of the past.

Inevitably we find ourselves in a situation where food and drink is consumed as quickly as possible - usually this starts at breakfast time; the kids have overslept and you had a 'late night' yesterday.

In our dash for school, work or the shops often our first meal will consist of two cups of coffee, toast, margarine and jam.

Lunch time sees the situation become worse as fast food outlets are besieged by the hungry mobs seeking the daily dose of burgers, fries and pastries!

The long term consequence of these habits can be seen in the number of people who feel listless; are sick, feeling 'off-colour', or who are continually constipated.

Chapter 6

By commencing your day with fresh vegetable juices you can make an excellent start to the process of removing the poisonous toxins, that have built up over the years, from your body. By adding just half a cap of 'liquid green chlorophyll' (made by Swisse) you add a nice mint flavour but also increase your intake of this important trace element.

JUICES - OTHER COMBINATIONS

There are many other variations for consuming vegetable juices. Here are just a few:

'STARTER'

6 carrots
2 sticks celery
2 slices beetroot
4 slices cucumber
2 broccoli heads
1 apple
1 handful lettuce

'LOOKING GOOD'

4 carrots
3 sticks celery
1 small handful parsley
plus a small amount of lemon juice

'ACHE-FIXER'

2/3 celery juice
1/3 apple juice

'REFRESHER'

4 carrots
2 sticks celery
1 handful lettuce
1 apple

Chapter 6

'ENTERTAINER'

This is a nice drink to give your guests - and not frighten them away!

> 4 carrots
> 2 sticks celery
> 1 apple, plus a teaspoon of honey

'THE CHAMPION'

> 7 carrots
> 3 sticks celery
> 1 apple
> 2 slices of beetroot
> 2 broccoli heads
> 1 hand full English spinach
> 1 hand full lettuce
> 1 small hand full parsley
> 4 slices cucumber
> 2 slices capsicum

JUICES FOR SPECIFIC DISORDERS

Vegetables, depending on their respective mineral and vitamin content, may assist in the case of specific disorders:

Acne
>   Carrots, spinach, celery, cucumber

Arthritis
>   Celery, cucumber, carrot

Blood Builder
>   Beetroot is wonderful as a blood builder

Blood Pressure
>   Celery and parsley; celery and cucumber

Constipation
>Any vegetable juice will assist but combinations of carrot and spinach; cabbage plus beetroot will be of benefit

Gout
>Celery and cucumber; carrot and spinach; beetroot and ripe tomatoes

Nervous system
>Celery; lettuce; carrot and lettuce combined; radish; beetroot

Sore throat
>Celery (fruit juices will probably be best for sore throats and we look at fruits in the pages that follow)

ONE LAST WORD ON VEGETABLE JUICE

If you suffer from arthritis, I urge you to try this juicing programme. My arthritis, diagnosed in 1992, has now completely disappeared and I have no signs of ANY arthritis in any part of my body... unbelievable? TRY IT!

FRUITS

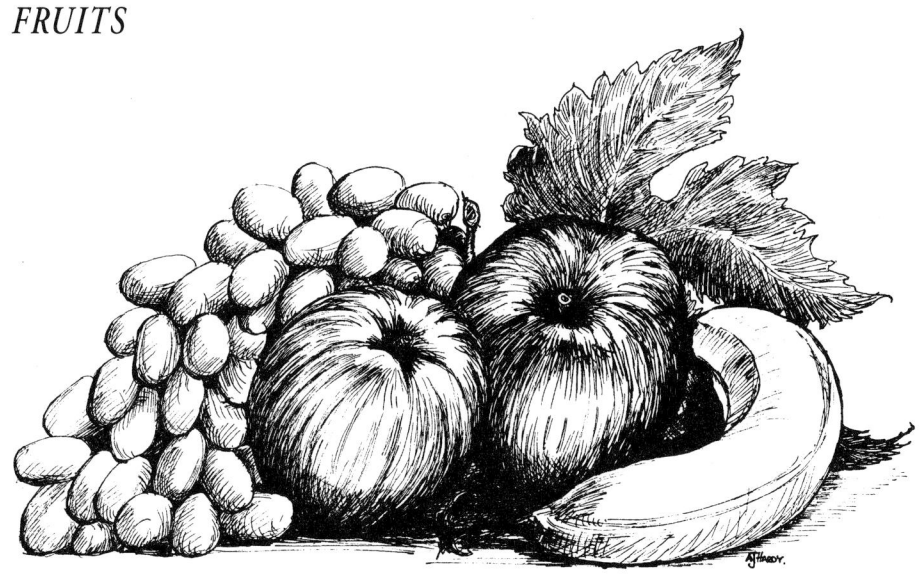

Chapter 6

The range of fruits in Australia is of course enormous. We are indeed fortunate that we have access to such variety and quality of these fresh fruits.

Fruit once juiced does remove fibre, making it easier for the essential nutrients to enter the bloodstream, so therefore it is ideal to also introduce raw fruit to your food intake, if you require the added benefit of fibre.

Personally I now enjoy fruit so much, I prefer to juice only rock melons (or cantaloupe) and enjoy the other fruits in their raw state as a fruit salad.

My favourite fruits are listed below:

Rock melon (cantaloupe)

Rock melon is rich in calcium, phosphorous, magnesium, plus it has vitamins A, B1, B2, B3 and C. It also is a good 'flusher' of waste from the body. It is probably best not to mix any other fruit with melons and besides they taste great on their own. We add a very small slice of raw ginger to provide a slight tang.

My wife and I enjoy 2 large glasses each of fresh rock melon juice every evening around 5-6 pm.

OTHER FRUITS

All other fruits are, in our household, eaten fresh and whole. I usually take fresh fruits to work and eat a large fruit salad as a mid afternoon snack.

Banana

Rich in potassium and an alkaline forming food, bananas contain all 6 essential vitamins. An excellent food, but for something different, try a banana smoothie by blending 1 large banana with ice cold soy milk - it's delicious.

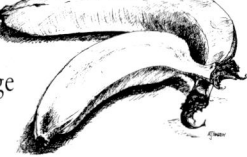

Apple

Apples contain many if not most of the essential minerals and vitamins we require. Apples also help maintain healthy skin, hair and teeth. 'An apple a day' really does 'help keep the Doctor away!'

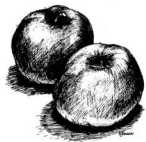

Grapes

Grapes can help in reducing blood acid levels, can assist with lowering blood pressure, assisting the liver and in the easing of arthritic pain. Grapes are high in potassium, magnesium, calcium and vitamins A, B & C.

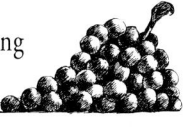

Strawberries

Wonderful in a fruit salad - both in colour and nutritional value - but wash them well before eating.
Strawberries are high in vitamin C and potassium, phosphorous and calcium.

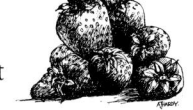

Kiwi Fruit

Our friends in New Zealand must have done something right - these delicious little fruits contain high levels of vitamin C plus essential elements such as magnesium and potassium.

Peach

Actually, an ideal fruit to juice - thick and creamy - it is also excellent in a fruit salad and is rich in vitamin A.

Oranges

Unfortunately these days it seems so much easier to pick up a bottle or carton of orange juice from the supermarket, rather than juice up fresh oranges.

Unfortunately, most commercial juices have been pasteurised, hence killing off the essential enzymes and also destroying most of the vitamin C.

Natural oranges can be juiced easily or eaten whole.

Chapter 6

A TYPICAL DAILY DIET

To provide an idea of just how simple and nutritional a fresh foods diet can be, I have listed two examples from a daily diet that I now follow:

Day 1 (weekday)	Early morning	4-5 glasses of fresh vegetable juice
	Mid morning	A handful of almonds and/or dates
	Lunch	1 or 2 whole-grain (preferably rye) rolls; fresh avocado as a spread (instead of butter and mayonnaise) and filled with salad. (The avocado adds a lovely moist creamy taste and blends well with the salads such as lettuce, cucumber, beetroot and carrot... and don't listen to anyone who says that avocado is high in cholesterol, it just isn't true as cholesterol can only be found in animal foods - not from the plant kingdom.)
	Mid afternoon	Fresh fruit salad made from 4 or 5 different raw fruits. Wash all fruit thoroughly prior to preparation.
	Early evening	2 glasses fresh rock melon (cantaloupe) juice
	Dinner	Vegetable and tofu lasagne

The actual recipe for vegetable and tofu lasagne follows:

VEGETABLE & TOFU LASAGNE

Lasagne can be prepared a day ahead; keep covered, in refrigerator. Lasagne can be frozen for a month. Cooked packaged lasagne can be used; you will need 150g (9 sheets) of wholemeal lasagne noodles.

- 1 tablespoon oil (preferably cold pressed olive oil)
- 2 medium onions, chopped
- 2 cloves garlic, crushed
- 2 medium carrots, chopped
- 2 large sticks celery, chopped
- 1 medium red pepper, chopped
- 200g mushrooms, chopped
- 6 medium tomatoes, peeled, chopped
- 2 tablespoons tomato paste
- 1/4 cup chopped fresh basil
- 1/4 cup chopped fresh parsley
- 3/4 cup soft tofu
- 300g fresh wholemeal lasagne noodles
- 1/4 cup stale wholemeal breadcrumbs
- 1 tablespoon grated parmesan cheese

Heat oil in large saucepan, add onions, garlic, carrots, celery and pepper, stir over medium heat for about 5 minutes (or microwave on HIGH for about 5 minutes) or until onions are soft. Add mushrooms, stir over medium heat for 1 minute (or microwave on HIGH for 1 minute). Stir in tomatoes, paste and herbs, bring to boil, reduce heat, cover, simmer for about 15 minutes (or microwave on HIGH for about 5 minutes) or until vegetables are tender. Remove from heat.

Beat tofu in small bowl until smooth, add 1/4 cup of the tofu to vegetable mixture, mix well.

Chapter 6

Cut pasta into 6 rectangles measuring about 10cm x 26cm. Spread a third of the vegetable mixture into greased 20cm x 26cm ovenproof dish (2 litre capacity). Top with 2 sheets of pasta. Continue layering vegetable mixture and pasta, finishing with a layer of pasta.

Spread remaining tofu evenly over pasta, sprinkle with combined breadcrumbs and a little cheese. Bake in moderate oven for about 50 minutes or until golden brown (or microwave on HIGH for about 25 minutes).

Serves 4

Day 2 (weekend)	Morning	4-5 glasses of fresh vegetable juice
	Mid morning	1 bowl of oatmeal or maize porridge with banana and soy milk (add a little organic rice syrup as a sweetener if necessary.)
	Lunch	1 or 2 whole-grain (or preferably rye) rolls; fresh avocado as a spread (instead of butter and mayonnaise) and filled with salad.
	Mid afternoon	Fruit salad
	Early evening	2 glasses of rock melon juice
	Dinner	Potato-Crushed Lentil Hot Pot
	Late evening	Banana smoothie

A special note: some people, initially at least, find it almost impossible to drink five glasses of vegetable juice either in the morning or at anytime. Simply start with two glasses each morning and the benefits will still begin to show.

Later you can slowly increase your juice intake to a level that you can comfortably accommodate.

The actual recipe for Potato-Crushed Lentil Hot Pot follows:

POTATO-CRUSHED LENTIL HOT POT

Hot pot is best prepared close to serving time. Recipe unsuitable to freeze or microwave.

3/4 cup red lentils	5 medium ripe tomatoes, peeled, chopped
5 medium potatoes	1 large vegetable stock cube, crumbled
1 tablespoon oil (olive oil)	1 cup water
2 medium onions, chopped	2 tablespoons tomato paste
2 medium carrots, chopped	2 tablespoons chopped fresh parsley
3 sticks celery, chopped	15g butter, melted
3 cloves garlic, crushed	1/4 teaspoon paprika
1 teaspoon curry powder	

Add lentils to large saucepan of boiling water, bring to boil, reduce heat, simmer, uncovered, for 10 minutes; drain well. Boil, steam or microwave potatoes in their skins until tender.

Heat oil in large saucepan, add onions, carrots, celery and garlic, stir over medium heat for about 5 minutes or until onions are soft. Stir in curry powder, cook for 1 minute. Add tomatoes, stock cube, water and paste, bring to boil, reduce heat, cover, simmer for 10 minutes. Stir in parsley and lentils; spoon into large ovenproof dish (8 cup capacity).

Slice potatoes, arrange over lentil mixture. (Brush potatoes, arrange over lentil mixture.) Brush potatoes with butter, sprinkle with paprika. Bake in moderate oven for about 45 minutes or until lightly browned.

Serves 4.

Both recipes shown above were supplied with the courtesy of 'The Australian Women's Weekly' who allowed the printing of the recipes from the book 'Vegetarian Cooking'[8].

I have mentioned almonds, and when you are travelling or going out, you may like to carry a supply in your car. Almonds are an alkaline food (other nuts are mostly acid foods) and are rich in potassium and have very little fat. Apart from having a delicious taste, almonds are a great snack that is actually good for you!

CHAPTER 7

— MEDITATION —

THE POWER OF A PEACEFUL MIND

Prior to 1993, I firmly believed that the only people who meditated wore orange clothes, sat cross-legged in the forest and chanted some strange words while playing with beads!

In fact, people from all walks of life - including leading business people, famous athletes and sports heroes - meditate. But what exactly is meditation and what are we trying to achieve by meditating?

We think nothing of resting our physical self each night - but our minds continue to work at '100kms an hour - non-stop'.

Meditating is not some complicated, mysterious ritual, but a simple process by which we are able to provide our minds with the opportunity to rest - and to release stress, anxiety and other mental activities which can often lead to serious illness.

Chapter 7

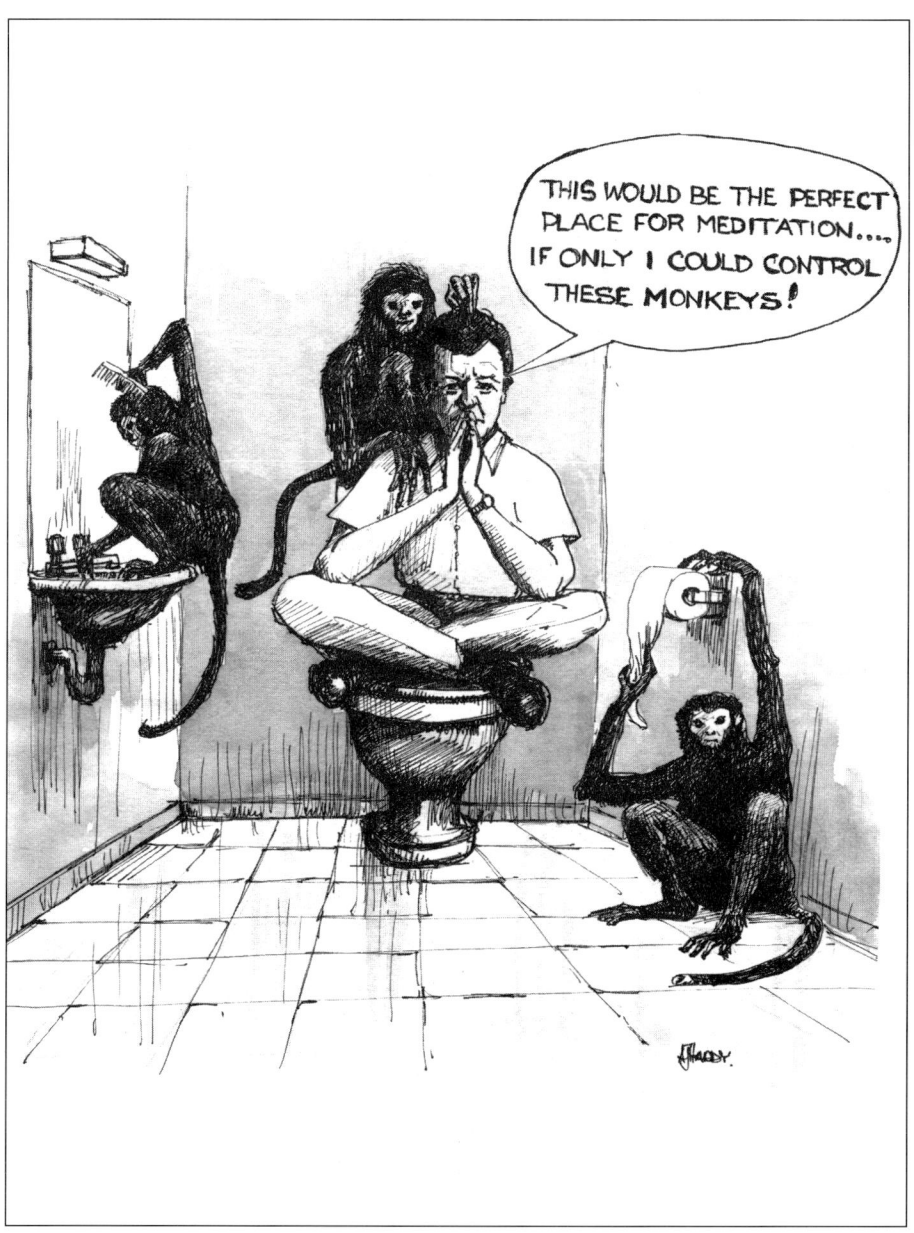

Chapter 7

THE 'MONKEY MIND'

Several years ago, I embarked on my first visit to a Buddhist Monastery - just south of Perth in Western Australia.

Whilst speaking with the Abbot (the Head Buddhist Monk), I asked him the inevitable question: 'Just what is meditation and what is one supposed to be doing or trying to achieve while meditating?'

It was then I was told about the 'Monkey Mind'.

'You see,' he explained, 'most Western minds are just like the monkey in the trees; always swinging from tree to tree, running here, jumping there... never taking the time to stop on one branch and resting a while because, if he did, he may have noticed how beautiful that particular tree was, and that it was laden with fruit to replenish and nourish its body.'

The analogy was as profound as it was simple. Meditation was or is nothing more than providing the opportunity and environment for the mind to rest - to take away stress, to put aside all worries and to spend time within one's own self.

A SIMPLE TEST

If you think it is ridiculous to suggest that you have a 'monkey mind', try this simple test.

Sit quietly in a dimly lit room. Be comfortable in a chair with your shoes off. Note the time and then close your eyes and think of nothing for 60 seconds...

Probability is that within 20 seconds, you are planning for today's activities; thinking about something that happened the other day, or just remembered something you had meant to do... our 'monkey mind' is alive and well and busy swinging from tree to tree.

The truth is - it is (initially) very hard to sit with a 'blank' mind for any amount of time, let alone a whole 60 seconds!

Why? Because ever since our birth, we have allowed our mind to take control of our thoughts and actions. We have allowed our mind to be like a petulant child, running around with no controls, direction or discipline.

Chapter 7

So throughout meditation, you can simply and harmoniously teach your mind to be quiet; to relax and allow itself to heal and repair the body.

Once you have mastered the art of settling the mind (and getting the 'monkey' to stay on one branch for a while), it is quite easy to introduce thought patterns that can stimulate the body's nervous and 'message' systems.

JUST HOW POWERFUL IS OUR MIND?

Over 35 years ago, then British neurophysicist, W Grey Walter, said that it would take at least 10 billion electronic cells to build a facsimile of the brain of a human. In his inspiring book 'Physco-Cybernetics[9]', Max Maltz correctly observes how 'we marvel at the awesome (power) of interceptor missiles which can compute in a flash the point of interception of another missile and 'be there' at (exactly) the correct instant to make contact.'

Yet (using my own example) we think nothing of watching a batsman hitting two or more runs in a game of cricket.

In order to have hit 'the two runs', his brain had less than quarter of a second to compute the speed of the ball from the bowler, its wind direction, the curvature of the fall, initial velocity and at the point of hitting the ball, sending a message to the legs, arms and feet, calculating how many runs can be taken, remembering to turn and run back. His computer compares this information with previous data ('experience') and makes these decisions. And we call this 'just hitting two runs'!

The human brain really is a most wondrous thing!

So imagine if we could access just a small fraction of this amazing computer to send it healing messages - remembering that the nervous system cannot tell the difference between an imagined experience and a real experience[10].

It simply reacts accordingly to what you think or imagine to be true.

Once again, remember that meditation is not some complex mystical rite performed by eastern 'witch doctors' - it is simply the art of bringing the mind to a restful and quiet state, so that we can then introduce chosen thought patterns and messages.

Chapter 7

CREATIVE VISUALISATION

Once you have gained some practice with meditation, it is possible to introduce 'creative visualisation' into your meditation.

This is the ability to create thoughts of your desire and to visualise them during your meditation. It could be walking in a forest, being in a quiet place in your home or walking along a beautiful beach. It can also be more specific.

Many people have spoken of visualising their good white cells attacking and destroying their cancer cells, with considerable success.

I personally do not like the concept of 'killing' or 'destroying' any part of my body, preferring to have the cancer cells 'converted' into good healthy white cells, or have the tumor slowly shrink in size until it disappears.

THE VANISHING FRECKLE

The following brief story perhaps helps to illustrate the potential power of the mind :

All my life, I had a dark brown birthmark in the form of a 'Hutchinson' freckle (about the size of a ten-cent piece) just near the front and middle of my lower neck where the two collar bones meet.

Over the years, various doctors had examined this 'Hutchinson' freckle to ensure that it was not growing or becoming larger. It never did change in colour and remained dormant.

After commencing meditation, I decided to focus on this freckle for no other reason other than to practice my creative visualisation.

So during each meditation, I would visualise my white cells of the immune system coming up and 'massaging away' this brown mark.

I felt I had become quite good at the technique and one morning, while standing in the bathroom cleaning my teeth, I looked into the mirror and couldn't believe my eyes ... the

Chapter 7

entire freckle was gone! In disbelief, I called (my wife) Katherine and asked if she thought my 'Hutchinson' freckle was getting smaller.

She looked at my neck area, then with a bewildered look said 'Where is it? It's not there?'

After 40 plus years, the freckle was gone.

A week later, I visited my dermatologist and he too was (very) surprised to see what had happened. But like most doctors, there has to be a medical reason behind everything.

His explanation was that 'on occasions, the immune system can attack foreign objects such as tumours, and in my case, a 'Hutchinson' freckle - reducing or eliminating them completely'.

This, no doubt, is probably true but I was left wondering what stimulates the white cells to do this?

While I cannot conclusively say it was the meditation and creative visualisation that eliminated the freckle, I have no doubt in my mind as to what was the driving force that stimulated the immune system to bring about this 'small miracle'!

THE GREATEST TEST WAS YET TO COME

Deep down every person who is in remission from cancer dreads the day that they may find another lump - whether it be in their breast, lymph glands or wherever.

In late February '96, this is exactly what happened to me. It was over two years since being first diagnosed; I had grown to thoroughly enjoy my fresh food lifestyle, mastered meditation and was physically fit. A new lump under my arm WAS NOT what I expected!

Yet, sure enough, now under my right arm-pit was a lump located in the lymph system.

PANIC SETS IN

My first reaction was one of panic. 'Oh no. This just cannot be. Not after all I've done.'

Then I realised that 'all I had done' was the perfect preparation to deal with the possibility of such an event.

Chapter 7

I then made a major decision. I would defer a visit to my oncologist for just two weeks. During that time, I would maintain my diet, increase meditation and try to visualise the lump away.

I honestly believed my body was ideally placed - both mentally, physically and internally - to deal with this crisis. The meditation became quite deep and within two weeks, I had a 'feeling' that all would be okay.

By the beginning of the third week, the lump had indeed diminished considerably and it was then I visited my doctor. Upon examination, he felt the lump was 'not significant' and suggested no further action.

At the time of writing my first book, the lump had continued to diminish and I continue to be in excellent health - still drinking fresh juices and meditating twice daily!

A special note here, that the purpose of this story is to demonstrate the power of the mind and the great advantages of meditation and diet. Under normal circumstances I would always recommend a patient refers him/herself to their doctor immediately when any such 'problem' arises.

So, therefore, it is important to remember that the many concepts discussed in this book are meant to complement existing medicine - Not replace it!

MEDITATION – *GETTING STARTED*

There are many forms of meditation and many ways of learning this ancient art of mind relaxation.

Libraries, Cancer Associations and book shops all have excellent literature on the subject. Most Buddhist temples and monasteries have monks who can also teach you meditation if you are well enough to visit.

When asked 'just how long will it take before I gain some benefit from meditation?' I often reply, 'Usually within 1-2 minutes !'

Such is the power of meditation that the benefits are, of course, almost instantaneous.

Chapter 7

SUPERVISED MEDITATION FIRST

It is not unusual that when people first start meditation, anger and/or negative feelings may start to emerge. Tears will quite often flow as the body finally has the opportunity to release all those hidden feelings and stress.

While not essential, sometimes it may be advisable to take up meditation in a supervised forum - particularly if you feel very stressed, hurt or confused.

An appropriately trained leader will understand your reactions and can provide assistance when and if necessary.

A SIMPLE TECHNIQUE

Following is a very simple alternative technique you may like to try:

Step 1

- Find a quiet room, preferably dimly lit where you can sit comfortably without being disturbed. (I found a wonderful location at our home which was away from the kids, the rabbit, the mice and the dog... in my car with the garage door closed!)

- Take off your shoes, place your watch so you can take a glance at the time when necessary.

- Let's aim for an initial meditation period of 20 minutes.

Step 2

- Focus on the breath flowing in and out of your nose, and as you do start to count slowly from 10 down to one.

- Once you have done this, then count from 10 down to 2.

- Then from 10 down to 3.

- Once you have reached a point whereby you have counted from 10 down to 9 you cannot go any further.

- Now quietly repeat an affirmation that suits you best. It may be simply:

  > 'May I be well'
  > 'May I be happy'
  > 'May I progress'

- Repeat this affirmation over and over - slowly; let your breath take its natural course.

- During this time, you will almost certainly notice your mind starting to 'wander all over the place'. This is quite normal, so just quietly return to the meditation each time this occurs.

Step 4

- Once you feel you have reached 20 minutes, open one eye and check your watch. If you still have some time to go, simply close your eyes and continue on.

- At the end of the meditation, take two more long slow breaths and slowly open your eyes, stretch and feel wonderful.

STRAY THOUGHTS

As mentioned earlier, almost certainly, when first starting meditation, you will find your mind will wander off in all sorts of directions. This is NORMAL - and you should NOT become frustrated or angry with yourself when this occurs, as over time you will teach your mind to settle down and to be quite focused on the meditation.

When during your count-down you find yourself thinking about what you have to do tomorrow, or yesterday's argument (or whatever), simply bring your mind back to the meditation (if necessary just start counting from 10 to 2 again).

No doubt your mind will wander off again. It's okay; just bring it back - slowly, nicely and without any annoyance. Meditation is meant to be a most natural and enjoyable activity - let it be that way.

After a while, your mind will be come accustomed to being focused and will not wander off quite so much.

Chapter 7

GUIDED MEDITATION

Some people find undertaking meditation alone and unaided difficult. There are a number of excellent cassette tapes available which will guide you through the meditation (hence the name 'Guided Meditation').

The meditations last from 20-40 minutes and all you need is a tape recorder - a 'walkman' tape deck with ear phone is ideal.

Remember, meditation is not some magical trick. Give it time and enjoy meditation as a time of day JUST FOR YOU! This is a time when you can 'go away' to any special place you desire; relax and to let your mind become quiet.

After a time meditation will become one of the most powerful tools available to you - it will become a part of your daily life.

If you can get your partner or friend to join you in your meditations all the better - you will feel the extra energy in the room!

'MIS'-GUIDED MEDITATION

One mistake that can be easily made is to assume that by 'simply closing my eyes and forcing myself to relax and remove all thoughts I can produce some magical change'.

People who approach meditation in this way are inevitably disappointed - and often feel even more stressed than before they started to meditate.

The objective of meditation is to be in the 'present moment' - without reflecting on yesterday or being concerned about tomorrow or even later today.

Give your mind the opportunity to become peaceful and calm. It will then evolve a process of eliminating concerns, worries and other thoughts.

Chapter 7

TRANSCENDENTAL MEDITATION (T.M.)

Transcendental Meditation (known simply as 'T.M.') was introduced to us by a mutual friend - Megan Bates - and, having meditated for over three years, we find T.M. both simple and highly effective.

'T.M.' works on the principle of two meditation periods each day (of 20 minutes) and the use of a 'mantra'.

For those who feel that they would like to experience and understand more about advanced meditation techniques, then 'T.M.' can prove very successful. Both Katherine and I now enjoy the 'T.M.' method of meditation twice daily.

'LEAKY' THE SHEEP

Meditation can also bring some very special moments, and such a moment occurred recently while Katherine and I were visiting a farm (some 200km south of Perth) owned by friends Geoff and Ronnie Willis.

On the first morning I decided to take advantage of the beautiful weather – cool and clear – and meditate on a ridge overlooking a small lake and stream.

It was 5.40am and I found a nice large stone upon which to sit. As the sun made its appearance over the distant hill I commenced what was going to be a very peaceful meditation.

Ten minutes later, with eyes closed and my mind in a still and quiet state, I became aware of a 'presence' very close to me. A short time later the feeling became so strong I slowly turned my head towards the 'presence' and opened my eyes only to find myself nose to nose with a very large sheep (ram).

Refusing to be flustered, I quietly looked into those big dark eyes and took the only course of action available...

'Excuse me' I quietly said feeling rather stupid, 'go away as I am meditating!'

Chapter 7

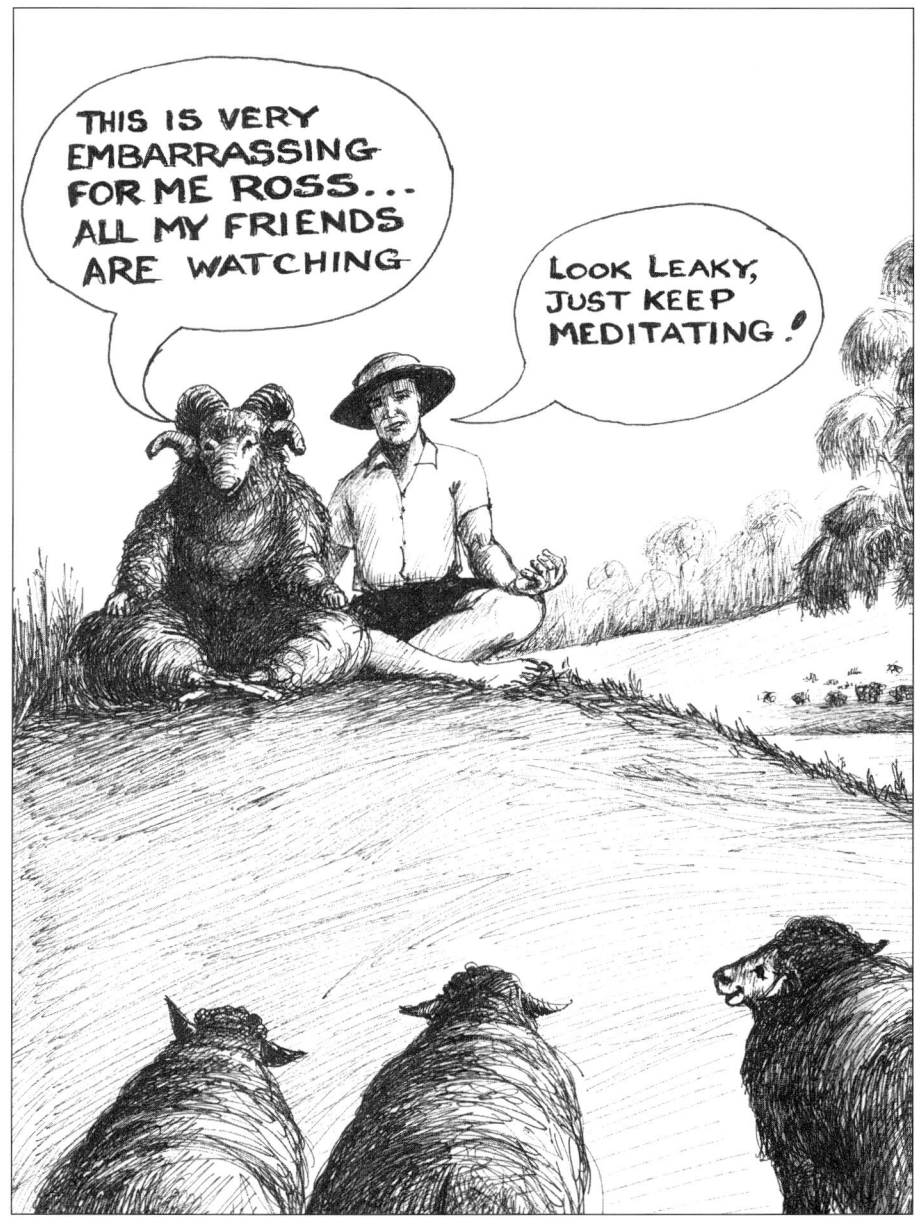

Chapter 7

Well, the sheep (whose name was later revealed as 'Leaky' – due to a urinary infection!) didn't go away, preferring to share my meditation and the peaceful energy that was surrounding us.

I must say, that the breath of an Australian sheep is not something I would get excited about!

ENJOYING TODAY

Through your meditation you can slowly learn the wonderful concept of how to truly 'live for today!'

Our lives are so busy planning for this, planning for that, worrying about tomorrow and agonising over some event that occurred yesterday, that we forget how to simply enjoy and embrace what it is we are doing today - or right now.

So when you are next washing the dinner plates, for example, and your mind is 'miles away', just look at what it is you are doing and concentrate on the task at hand.

Surely you will start to appreciate each day as it really is.

I always remember John Lennon's famous words, *'Life is something that happens while you are busy making other plans...'*.

CHAPTER 8

– PHYSICAL FITNESS –

It is always preferable to complement good diet and meditation with some physical activities.

Personally, I have enjoyed swimming for many years and I currently swim 3-4 kilometres per week.

It is important to remember that it is the lymph glands that collect all the toxins and poisons from your body. Unfortunately, the lymph glands need stimulation beyond that which nature provides. Therefore exercise provides the stimulation so very necessary to clean and move the toxins from the lymph glands and out of the body.

TAKE TIME FOR EXERCISE

Everyone should exercise. It helps the body maintain strong bones and improves the heart rate and circulation. Since exercising my heart rate (resting) has dropped from 72 to 61 beats per minute. Doesn't sound much does it? But say if I told you that, in order to keep me alive, every year my heart now pumps 5.78 million times less than before.

Most people desire to undertake some form of exercise, yet inevitably everyone seems too busy or under too much pressure to have time to exercise. If we could allocate just 1% of our time each week for exercise, we could be fit for life!

This 1%, or 100 minutes per week, could be carried out by swimming, jogging or simply

Chapter 8

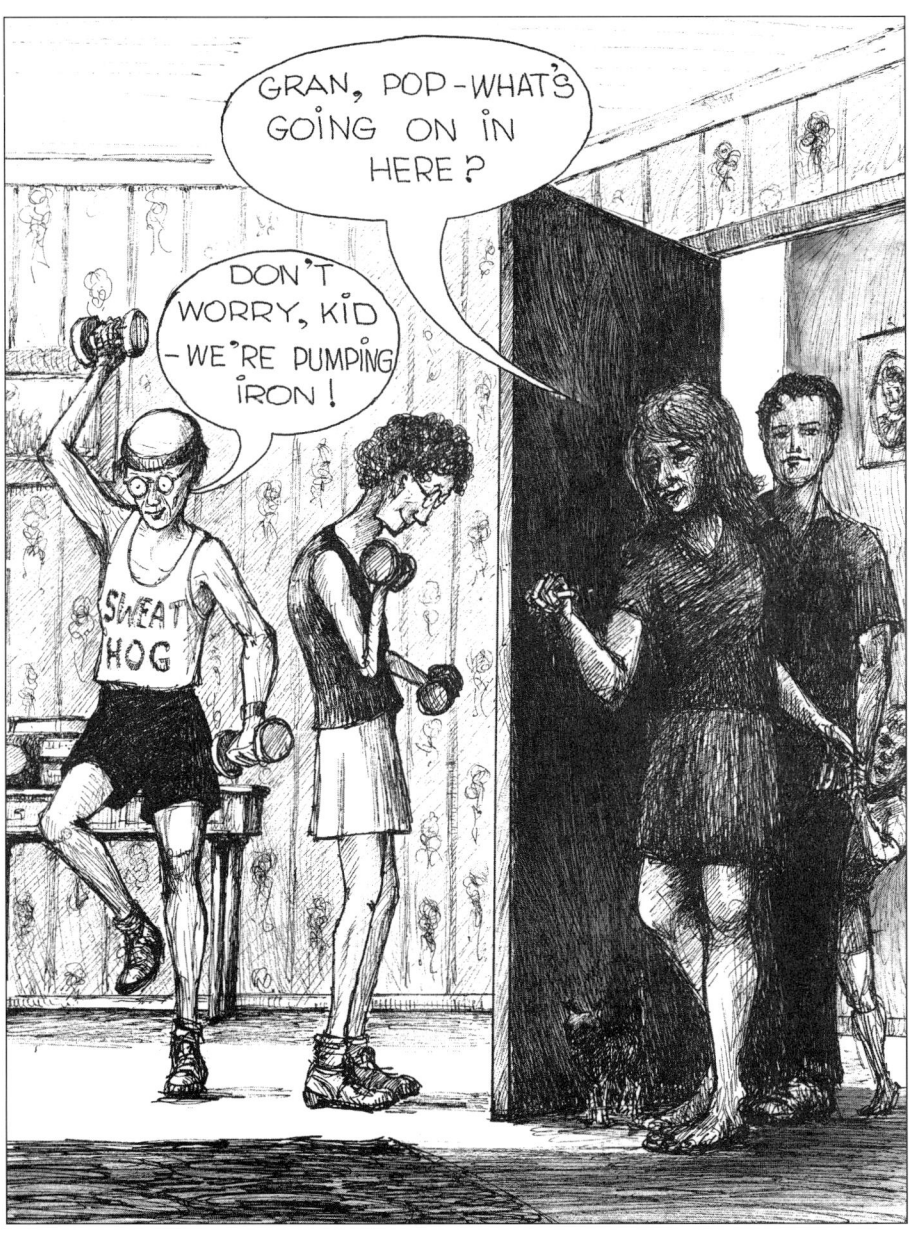

Chapter 8

walking. Katherine and I regularly walk - along with Penny (our dog), and in the process breath the morning air, notice the beautiful white-gum trees in our park and meet lots of nice people.

The ancient Chinese art of Tai Chi and Qi Gong are also very good forms of physical exercise, with the added bonus of calming the mind.

As our population becomes older there is ongoing concern about degenerative diseases such as osteoporosis.

Evidence is now strongly suggesting that a high animal protein diet and a sedentary lifestyle are the major causes of bone disease.

So when considering exercise also try to include weight resistant activities to ensure your muscles and bones are exercised.

The concept of grandfather 'pumping iron' at the local gym may sound hilarious but in a controlled and modified programme it may be the best thing he could do!

Physical exercise will not, on its own, cure anyone from cancer. It will, however, contribute to an improved sense of well-being and allow your body to be healthier and fitter - and be in a better position to assist in the healing process.

CHAPTER 9

– SPIRITUAL –

A Higher Power

Your own beliefs and religion will provide you with your own answers on this subject.

I was born as an Anglican Christian but like many Australian baby-boomers it has been a number of years since I last visited my local church.

Yet I still possess an extremely strong feeling of 'closeness' with my God.

Yes, I do believe in a 'higher power' and find it very helpful to complete my morning and evening meditation with a silent prayer whereby I thank God for giving me another beautiful day on this incredible planet.

If you are a regular member of the local church or religious group you may find it helpful to discuss your feelings and progress with the religious leader of your choice.

If you don't attend a religious centre, do what I have done and take just a few minutes to give thanks each day and reaffirm your commitment to becoming well again.

At the conclusion of each meditation (morning and evening), take time for a small prayer and you will find this a very lovely way to ease your way back into everyday activity.

Chapter 9

The emotional Connection

Whilst discussing spirituality, we should also look at the connection between cancer and past or present emotional issues.

There is only a limited amount of scientific evidence to support such a connection, however, for many people cancer is a time when they must face emotional issues in order to allow complete healing to take place. Unfortunately this issue is sometimes far too difficult to confront as it often requires a complete re-evaluation of one's own life and values.

People (including me) who can never say 'no' and are always there to 'help out', or feel it is their duty to take on the total responsibility of the entire family for example, are often those who eventually face life-threatening diseases such as cancer... but why?

As occurred in my own life, I believe that by placing unrealistically high expectations upon one's self, combined with a deep-seated need to please everyone, creates an environment whereby the body and soul begins to look for a socially acceptable way out of this unwinnable game!

Anger, hurt and bitterness can also cause great damage and create a dangerous 'mind-set' along with considerable unhappiness and a sense of being alone. Many cancer patients with whom I have associated, have benefited enormously from having worked through a process of learning how to love themselves first and then introduce the concept that 'I'm OK'.

In creating a holistic approach to your recovery from cancer it is most important to consider these issues. This can often be difficult to do and therefore counselling can often be very helpful. Emotional issues should, however, be faced as the other forms of healing, to which I have already referred, can only be fully effective when they work in synergy with emotional healing.

Dr Daniel Benor [14] in a recent address had this to say, 'Healing is the ability to let out anger and negativity but at the same time to forgive and accept the inevitable frailties of others, and even more difficult, of one's self.'

I urge you to read this statement again for it is indeed profound.

CHAPTER 10

– REIKI –

The Ancient Japanese Art of Energy Transfer

During the period of treatment and subsequent research into this book, I was astounded at the enormous quantity of cures, solutions, potions and alternative medicines being promoted to people suffering from cancer.

It is little wonder people become confused!

Because of the wide range of options, I chose only those detailed in this book ... 'sticking with the tried and proven methods' was my belief.

I should relate to you, however, about my introduction and experience with an ancient Japanese art of healing through energy renewal using the hands. This practice is known as 'Reiki'.

Once taught, the concept is quite simple in that energy can be transferred through one's hands onto the body of oneself or another person (or any animal for that matter!)

Chapter 10

A BRIEF HISTORY

The simple concept of hands-on energy renewal was first discovered - in fact re-discovered - by a Dr Mikao Usui (who lived in Kyoto, Japan) just over 100 years ago.

After an exhaustive search as to how the ancient people healed by using their hands, Usui was finally able to translate an obscure Sanskrit manuscript which explained the art of Reiki.

After experimenting, he was astonished at the results, including not only healing but developing a calm and peaceful disposition, reduction of stress and nervous tension and reduction in muscle pain.

Unlike the other oriental arts of Qi Gong and Tai Chi, the energy flow generated through Reiki has its origins externally - entering via the head.

Reiki was introduced to the Western world in the early 1970s by Hawayo Takata. Mrs Takata had been a student of Mikao Usui's successor Dr Chujiro Hayashi.

Reiki has now spread throughout the world and has a large following in Australia. Some practise Reiki professionally while others, such as myself, simply enjoy its enormous benefits by itself.

I had first encountered Reiki while visiting the Cancer Support Association in Cottesloe. I was introduced to one of their carers, Cathy Brown, who provided a one hour session of Reiki.

It was fascinating that her left hand - which was placed above the shoulder where my tumor had been initially removed - started to shake quite strongly, during the Reiki session.

Cathy commented that this particular area of my body was drawing-in tremendous levels of healing energy, thus prompting her to ask me why this would be so. I was then able to explain about the secondary tumor. Likewise, another carer at the C.S.A., Doreen, would notice her left hand vibrate vigorously while applying Reiki to me.

Chapter 10

OUR FIRST REAL LIFE REIKI EXPERIENCE

In January 1995, our family was holidaying in the Kalbarri National Park (150km north of Geraldton, Western Australia). This is a magnificent area with towering gorges, vividly contrasting coloured hills and cliffs dropping several hundred metres to the Murchison River below.

While the park is quite stunning, the walk (there is no access to motor vehicles) into the gorges takes over 1 hour and in the middle of summer, with temperatures around 44°C, the task can be extremely challenging.

We had waited four days for the weather to cool a little, but this was not to be, so on our final day we decided to proceed with the tour of this area which resembles a mini-version of America's Grand Canyon!

All went well, until at the end of the morning when we returned to the tour bus, after trekking for an hour from the river over the gorges and back to the roadside in blistering heat.

One couple had taken their 10 year old son along and upon reaching the bus, it was apparent he had been affected with sunstroke. Very distressed, he screamed that he felt his head was going to 'burst'; he was hot, flushed and the cool towels did not seem to help.

My wife, Katherine, who had been practising Reiki for only nine months, quietly applied her hands to the boy's head as he sat in the bus, obviously in considerable pain.

Within two minutes his crying stopped and he became calm, commenting, 'What are you doing... it feels nice... please keep your hands there'.

Katherine maintained the Reiki during the 50 minute drive back to the township, where upon the boy - now feeling much better - was taken to the Doctor for observation.

Until this time, I had been somewhat cautious about Reiki, but after witnessing this incident I decided to complete a Reiki training programme, similar to the course taken by Katherine nine months earlier.

Chapter 10

The course took three days and I now (selfishly) use Reiki on myself while lying in bed by just simply placing the hands on strategic locations around the chest and stomach. I stopped applying Reiki while watching television because inevitably it would put me to sleep.

Today, my wife continues her voluntary work providing Reiki to many people who seek its benefits, while I continue to use Reiki for my own benefit.

I must comment, though, that animals react marvellously to Reiki. Our pet rabbit and young dog will sit quietly in our lap whilst Reiki is applied to their back and stomach. Instinctively, the pets seem to know that this 'hands-on' activity is something much more than just a friendly pat on the back.

Therefore, I leave it to you to make your own judgement. Reiki, however, does deserve your serious consideration.

CHAPTER 11

– VITAMINS –

Dr Ian Brighthope, who is a fellow of the Australian College of Nutritional and Environmental Medicine says that *'in nature there are a wide variety of naturally occurring antioxidant mechanisms... A number of important proteins play key roles... including various antioxidant enzymes. Various trace elements act as cofactors to a number of these enzymes - including zinc, copper, manganese and selenium.'* [12]

In a perfect world, with good availability of natural foods, there should be no need to have vitamin supplements. Unfortunately we no longer live in a perfect world. In fact the air that we breath, the water we drink and the food we eat contains 'free radicals' (not the human-type who protest in the forest!) which can create havoc within our cell structure and cause a wider range of diseases including cancer.

Therefore we do need to take vitamin supplements - particularly those that act as anti-oxidants such as grape seed extract. Vitamin 'C' also assists greatly in the retention of iron.

The type of vitamins that you consume is also most important. Vitamin supplements need to be 'synergised', in much the same way as the vitamins found in natural fruit and vegetables, work in harmony with each other.

While I am reluctant to start recommending particular brands of vitamin supplements, a recently released brand known as Usana, and also the Pharma range have left me highly

Chapter 11

impressed with the level of quality control, synergy and potency achieved in their products.

So before starting to use vitamin supplements it is important to see a good Naturopath to ensure that your programme is well balanced and that you are not simply flushing $$$ of vitamins down the toilet every day!

A NOTE ABOUT SELENIUM

Selenium is a mineral which, after many years of fertilisers and pesticides being applied to our soils, has almost vanished.

Until I was diagnosed with cancer, I must admit to not even having knowledge about Selenium, other than knowing that it had some vague connection with healing sick animals and that farmers would use it on their stock.

Over the past 10 years, there has been mounting evidence that Selenium does play an important role in the prevention of various cancers.

Research in America has shown that selenium can reduce cancer mortality by as much as 50%[13] and has also been shown to improve the immune response in many other animal species.

Selenium deficiency also DECREASES the immune response.

People in low-Selenium areas (or countries) appear to experience greater risk of cancer than people in high Selenium countries[14].

Dr Ian Brighthope has stated that in his opinion *'Selenium is probably one of the **most** important trace elements in the overall consideration of antioxidant defence mechanisms'.*[15]

It is also reported that in New Zealand the human and animal populations have amongst the lowest selenium intakes in the world. The incidence of carcinoma of the colon is also the highest in the world, plus there is a very high rate of breast cancer. There may be a relationship between low selenium intake and these cancers.

Unfortunately in Australia, Selenium until just recently had been banned from retail sale.

Chapter 11

This has created a crazy situation whereby all farmers use selenium routinely to protect their animals, yet we mere humans require a prescription. It can now, however, be obtained without prescription from selected pharmacies or, alternatively, you can obtain Selenium tablets from New Zealand or South East Asia. Many of these tablets, incidentally are made... in Australia!

I have included details of Selenium in this book because of the evidence in favour of its uses. In addition, prominent Australian nutritionists also suggest there is a strong link between Selenium and the improvement in the recovery from cancers.

There is a good book available in most book-shops which should be compulsory reading for ALL people.

'Selenium - As a Food & Medicine'

by

Dr Richard A Passwaters
PIVOT Original Health Books
Keats Publishing Inc., Connecticut, USA

I leave it to you to decide - and as always discuss this with a Naturopath first.

CHAPTER 12

– LOOKING AHEAD –

Anyone who has lost a loved one or has experienced a life-threatening disease is only too well aware that amid the pain and suffering... life around you simply does go on.

And while your friends will eventually forget about the disease that so dramatically affected your life, cancer is something that you will never forget.

Even the most outgoing and optimistic people would probably admit that it is quite normal to have moments of doubt and anxiety - even four years on.

I have dealt with this situation by acknowledging that life is, indeed, a precious gift. That everyday is new and exciting, and therefore I will enjoy each day to my full ability because it is good to be alive TODAY.

I have also adopted a more 'easy going' approach to life... by not taking things quite so seriously. It is important to learn to laugh and smile a lot and to decide to be genuinely happy with one's life, as it is today. And don't take life too seriously!

I was recently asked a surprising - but very honest - question about the publication of this book. My friend cautiously asked 'what if, after publishing this book, you were to get sick again?'

For, although I intend to live a long and healthy life it is possible for the cancer to return.

Chapter 12

The reality is, however, that through practising and embracing the philosophy and programmes as outlined in this book, I have been able to enjoy a wonderful, healthy four years filled with a new inner peace and awareness. So no matter what the future holds, the fact remains that I enjoy and love life TODAY.

I have created an environment both emotionally, spiritually and physically whereby my entire 'body' is balanced.

When I look around me and see those people who have not only lived, but thrived with cancer, they often fit into the following grouping:

- They eat and drink sensibly and enjoy a diet that is rich in 'living' foods
- They meditate and have reduced stress
- They have developed a new spirituality
- They embrace life - and laugh a lot
- They have a total commitment to being alive and well
- They live for the 'moment'.

Even those people who eventually passed-over were able to enjoy a significantly improved quality of life and inner peace.

Last year while attending a cancer discussion group, I listened to one such lady named Helen Benham as she gave hope and encouragement to another lady who had just been diagnosed with cancer.

Helen, who had endured some enormous challenges as a result of cancer affecting her life, was perhaps one of the best examples of how people could successfully live with cancer.

Chapter 12

After listening to her words I went home and searched through some papers and found the following small piece written by William Aden White. I would like to now share this with you:

'I am not afraid of tomorrow,
for I have seen yesterday
and I love today'

After reading these beautiful words, I paused for a moment, and asked myself 'Does this really reflect how I now feel about my life?'

I smiled quietly to myself and then said out loud

'Yes it does ... it really does!'

THE END

CHAPTER
13

– *SOURCE AND REFERENCE* –

1. Cancer Support Association:
   80 Railway Street, Cottesloe, Western Australia 6011

2. Dr Barbada Anderson Ph.D. Ohio State University. Research Programme 1997

3. Dr Max Gerson 'A Cancer Therapy; Results of Fifty Cases' 1958
   Totality Books, California USA

4. 'The Pursuit of Life' by Lai Chiu-Nan Ph.D.
   Published by Lapis Lazuli Pte Ltd Singapore

5. 'The Truth About Milk Consumption'... Dr Shu-Hui Chiang
   'Lapis News' 4th issue Oct-Dec 1997

6. Journal of the National Cancer Institute (USA) June 1993

7. 'Juicing for Health' by Julie Stafford; Penguin Books Australia Ltd
   Book published 1994

8. 'Vegetarian Cooking' - The Australian Women's Weekly
   ACP Publishing Pty Ltd 1989

9. 'Physco-Cybernetics' by Max Maltz Page 23-26
   Book published 1960

10   Schrauzer, G. White D. & Schneider C. 1977

11   Dr Daniel Benor. 'Psychotherapy and Spiritual Healing'. Paper presented to the 'Body, Mind and Soul' conference, Melbourne, Australia. March 1998

12   Dr Ian Brighthope; Fellow Australian College of Nutritional and Environmental Medicine ... Paper September 1995

13   Journal American Medical Association. December 1996

14   'Selenium - As a food and medicine' Dr Richard Passwaters; Keats Publishing. 1980

15   Dr Ian Brighthope; Fellow Australian College of Nutritional and Environmental Medicine... Paper September 1995

- **SEMINARS**
- **GROUP MEETINGS**
- **CORPORATE FUNCTIONS**
- **CLUBS ETC...**

The author of 'Living Simply with Cancer' (Mr Ross Taylor) provides interesting and challenging talks on the following subjects:

- 'Living with Cancer'*
- 'Reducing your chances of getting cancer and other life-threatening diseases'*
- 'No fat, no stress'
- 'How to do business without stress and without getting fat!'
- 'The myth about diets'
- 'Striving and thriving in the next century'

(* The author does not charge any fee for talks related to cancer) For more information about these talks contact:

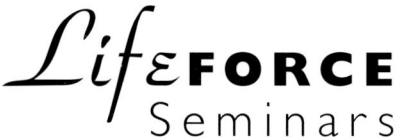

*Life***FORCE**
Seminars

Postal Address ~ PO Box 125 Greenwood Western Australia 6924
Telephone / Facsimile (61 8) 9448 1963 Email ~ ross@lifeforce.iinet.net.au